SEX, DRUGS AND NORTHERN SOUL

The Story

By Raymond Brown & Jason Tune

'One million people commit suicide every year'
The World Health Organization

Published by:
Chipmunkapublishing
PO Box 6872
Brentwood
Essex
CM13 1ZT
United Kingdom

http://www.chipmunkapublishing.com

Second edition Feb 2007

I've known Jason since he was about 11 years old at Kimberworth school. I had my first introduction to Jason when he was fighting with about 3 lads my age, I'm two years older than Jason and I stepped in to split things up. I never really had much to do with Jason apart from saying hello at school.

A few years later I'd gone in the forces and came home one weekend to be told by several people, J, as he was known had been looking for me all week but when I asked why, no one had dared ask as Jason had one bad reputation. Anyhow next thing Jason turns up and it was to thank me for helping him about 7 years before, and we've remained friends ever since.

That introduction just about sums Jason up as he never seems to forget anything. I hope this book Jason is doing is a great success as Jason has been through as many problems as anyone I know and somehow came out the other side as a great person whose main aim in life is to help others who are having similar problems to what he's been through.

 Good Luck Jason you deserve it pal

Denis Coleman
Chairman (Rotherham United Football Club)

Chapter 1: My Infancy

The icy wind meant more scarves wrapped tighter than ever. The darkness was descending fast with many an apprehensive look to the fast approaching rain. Listerdale Maternity Home, Ward 3, heard the first cry of one, Jason Tune.

The ward sister entered the relevant details. Boy, weight 10 pounds and counting, date Tuesday, the 28th.of November, year of our Lord 1964. Father's name: Patrick Gillott Tune. Mother's name: Anne Tune, address somewhere in the bowels of Rotherham town.

People nodded; doting Aunties cooed; sisters looked on in awe and an unrecognised sense of change. "Big, Int he?" "Should have picked him up by the nose, God bless him". And so the first day of my life passed.

"Well", said the sister, "I think that you can take him home. We can't afford the baby milk". "Mothers' milk will have to do". A quick change of the Trackies propelled me home to a typical two up, two down mid terrace house in 'sunny' Masbrough. So, thought I, life consists of tin baths and freezing outside toilets. The occasional visits to the corner shop for our daily bread and a packet of Park Drive cigarettes. The doting Aunties arrived every Sunday for a bit of snap and an hour of juicy gossip. In between 'Have you heard' and 'Well I never', I learnt to walk, talk and pee on my own. My sisters taught me to speak and my

Father taught me not to repeat what they taught me.

By the age of four I was the middle child of five. The family Tune whistled a song and departed for the luxury of a council house in the res-des area of Meadowbank, Lower Kimberworth, of course. Having an inside bath at least stopped my sisters from telling me that I would not grow up like them. Life was fun. The cry of "the wind has changed" meant everybody ramming rag filled sausages to the doors and handkerchiefs round the mouth. The gentle folk of Sheffield had a lot to answer for; offering their daily deposits. Rather ironic considering I lived close to the sewage works at Meadowbank. Perhaps the town planners were having a joke of their own. I doubt if any bank ever had that type of deposit. Not the best manure for the allotment.

Looking like a S.A.R.S riddled country was enough for my Father to change address once more. We moved up in the world: one street higher on the estate, to be precise. 'Posh them there Tunes', seemed to be the regular neighbourhood slag off. A corner house, with our own gate attached. Modern home improvement programmes could have learnt a thing or two. Contentment was using an attached toilet without listening to the chatter of other sitting residents. My kingdom became the street and beyond. Luxury was a quick nip to the 'chippy' on a Friday night for chips and scraps with heavy on the vinegar and light on the salt.

Sometimes, the daily patrol of my territory involved a visit to my Grandparent's. Gran's is a mixture of faded memories and half forgotten smells of home baking. Whenever my tummy was growling a quick 'hello Grandma' it was followed by a door wedge of the best dripping with a dash of 'Henderson's' to salivate the throat. Ten minutes after my goodbyes found me wiping my plate at home with a slice of bread (for mopping up purposes). No wonder the sight of me was always met with, "Big, int he". Living in a family where my Mother inevitably called each offspring by at least three names before the almost right one was applied, in a way pushed me towards my Grandparent's where I rapidly became the prince of the castle. "I am Captain of the ship", was my Granddad's favourite expression and I loved him all the more for it.

My quick ten minutes visits became thirty minutes and rising fast. When the Captain of the ship said 'you might as well move in' I arrived with my bedding, pack of cards, change of underwear and settled into life as number one cabin boy.

One day, my Grandma washed the back of my ears more vigorously than usual. I thought to myself, as it was not the third Sunday after Lent, what was going on. My National Health designer glasses were rammed over my head, shoes polished to perfection, "Ah, he'll do" from Cap'n, and off I was dragged. And, so, on the first day of school in September 1969, I found myself in an Infants class at Kimberworth Infant (and some say, corrective) School. I wondered why all the kids were crying for their Mothers or peeing on the floor. Ah well, I thought, it will be O.K. before I went home for lunch. Little did I realise that it meant every day and all day.

A very early but totally un-comprehended stigma befell me by break-time. The gallant three, as we thought we were, but known as 'the freebies' to others, were told that we had to queue up together for our lunch. Free school lunch was something that took a while for me to understand and hate. Of course, the food converter known as my stomach was not about to rebel.

"Hey, Tuney", a nondescript said, "Why dus thy wear specs then?" The truth be known was because I had a lazy left eye with a word that I could not spell to describe it. "Ah, don't know", was my reply. Immediately the Lower Kimberworth pack animal instincts kicked in and I had four days of constant, "Clarence, the cross-eyed lion". My Grandma taught me that everyone was important and all should be treated right. The baying audience had no idea of the hurt inside me.

One day, whilst walking to the establishment for the betterment of unreasoning urchins, a group of Ties as they were known (the big school kids) heard the daily prayers being chanted in my direction and changed the Kimberworth Book of Common Prayer to "Boss eyed B". I stood there in the middle of a co-ordinated word stoning ritual and thought to myself with an almost evangelical fervour that, one day, I would rule the group of Ties and become the local Robin Hood. Tune the Hood. Nice ring to it. I would give back to the verbal tyrants and defend my mates. Bugger the also-rans; I was not that soft a lad.

The pecking order in the Infants was sorted out very early. Big Bob, as he was known, was on the black part of the old school yard and I was the white king. The black part was tarmac for official school games and the white area was concrete for illicit games and general mayhem. Big Bob reigned supreme on the black part of the playground. Soon, the name Big Bob was dropped as fast as Big Bob was dropped by me. I became king of the black and whites. No name calling came my way, only a grudging respect from the numbers two, three, four, all the way to the ones who were not even classified.

At the age of five I had claimed my first title and my territorial rights of ownership were extended. However, I was not all about a well-connected slap in the head but more to do with the formation of friendships. Some of these have proved to stand the test of time. Big Bob became my right hand man and I dealt with whatever he managed to make a mess of. I felt like a vacuum cleaner cleaning up the rubbish that befell me. Usually, an introduction to my clenched hammer hand was sufficient for even the ones with no brain cells linked together.

Skelly, the name allocated by a generation of kids to the ever-patient teacher of the tribe, awarded me the prestigious title of chief book and class monitor. Of course, I was not aware of it immediately but there was a well functioning brain in my head and I found to my surprise and delight that I actually enjoyed the schoolwork.

My favourite party trick was to sing my number two times table. By the time my relatives were yawning in boredom I had rattled off the alphabet and my name spelt in big letters. As a reward for my enterprising academic achievements my Grandma began to take me to the weekly church jumble sale. Before the age of six I knew the insides of every local church and some beyond. Not for the glorification of the bloke called God who figured in most peoples conversations, "Oh my God". I was instructed to look through the keyholes to spy what was for sale and what was on offer. Poll position was often ours by half past five but the weekly gathering soon built up to frenzy. "Watch out", came the cry from Grandma, "It's the Hazelwood's". "She is a varmint that one. Get in there before them, I said". Six O'clock was inevitably the commencement of the entry scrum but look forward Tune was in there first and the prized pair of football boots was mine. By this time I was big enough to stuff my intended purchases up my armpit. I only intended to purchase them if I was caught. Any change I had left, or more to point not spent, was traded in for the biggest bag of sweets that I could buy. The agonies of whether I should have four blackjacks or six of them haunt me to this day.

So, seven O'clock found me hurtling home or should I say back to my Pirate Ship? The sheets pegged to the washing lines were my sails and the television masts my Jolly Roger. I knew that the Cap'n was waiting for his booty.

"What's for tea then, Granddad?" "An thy can go to thi muvvers for tea". I didn't mind as it meant some more food and a shared bottle of Ben Shaw's finest fizzy pop. This was my ale. It was to be a while before I was to taste proper beer but my imagination was good enough now. If my Dad was flush or had not called in for a quick pint on the way home we were treated to a bag of sugared almonds or even a big bag of Yorkshire mixtures. Special occasions were sherbet pips. At least it stopped the growling in my stomach. Talk about living life in an all-inclusive set-up. We had it first.

Up the hill, where my Grandparent's lived, I could hear the church bells ring out nine O'clock and that signalled my descent into the world where I was king and all I surveyed was mine. Dreams do come true but that was for the future. No roosters where I lived but the early morning call came instead from the Cap'n. "Thi teas ont table and tha can get thi sen up to school early for a change". Sure enough I did what I was told; gulped the tea and sneaked one last wedge of bread with whatever on it and dashed down the road to meet my sister Cheryl. She is eleven months older than me and she was now in her middle year at little Kimmy Infants. The school has always been known by this tag. I had changed places with Cheryl at my Grandparent's house. The Cap'n would often call her Topsy after the name of the latest fad in dolls at the time. She went back to my parents to share a bedroom and many rows with my oldest sister Marina. Amongst the siblings Marina was an awesome sight when she was demonstrating her position as number one child. Still is, now, but I dare not admit it. Cheryl would be like the family newspaper. She would disclose tittle-tattle and gossip on a daily basis. Information about all and sundry came my way. Often, I would not have a clue what she was on about and it was a long time later before I found out that she did not know either.

Our epic journey to school took us along the 'Lane'. One side was posh, that being the Kimberworth side. Across the lane was our end. We would cut through the allotments and call at Barrowclough's for an ice cream or penny lollypop. It was just someone's front room made into an impromptu shop selling bits and pieces to passing trade, mainly us. As we walked along more pirates would join our happy band and we would sail into the schoolyard for new adventures.

Cheryl, one day, announced that we, not her, were not going to school. We were to sail the seven seas and hoist the skull and crossbones. "Why?" I asked before I realised that I had questioned the first mate in a scurvy and disrespectful manner. Whilst I was enjoying my luck at not having my head bashed by my fellow pirate, she was explaining that the previous day she had stolen her teacher's special silver, really sharp... 'Be careful, children'... pencil sharpener. The Spanish inquisition had nothing on that afternoon's questioning. Cheryl dare not go back and face the gangplank and the teacher infested waters. "O.K", said I, wondering why my stomach was making odd purring noises. As time went on I had mixed feelings about the decision. Mainly because I was on free meals and I was missing my dinner. No food in our galley at the top of Meadowbank.

The next day I weighed anchor at headquarters and told them that Cheryl was sick. They must have thought I had been too as no request for a note was made. Thus, my life on the wild side was now a fact and not a quick 5 minute day dream, when my teacher was explaining the mechanics of the two times table. Now there is a thought: why did we have to sing it?

Dad at the time had just part exchanged his first car, a Mini with a go faster white stripe, for a Morris Minor with Walt Disney transfers emblazoned on every available surface. "Is that a bloody car or an advert? Scathingly remarked by peg leg, blue beard up the road. Once per week my Dad took a gang of us swimming to the main swimming baths in Rotherham. The journey was always over the newly built Tinsley viaduct. I always thought that he took us that way for the view from the bridge. It was only in my new life that my Dad finally admitted that he took us that way to avoid going through the town centre. A Guinness bottle label was still in use as a substitute car tax disc even then.

One day, Cheryl was asked to remove the transfers and clean the car for the princely sum of half a knicker (or 50p in toy town money). Poor bugger, she scrubbed and scrubbed for over three hours with much encouragement from the assembled troops. Better than television that was. "It's my money", she yelled. "No bloody chance" was the universal chorus and she was whisked into the nearest sweet shop with strict instructions to the proprietor that she was paying. No growling that afternoon. Wagging was forgiven but the thrill of cocking a snoop at authority secretly thrilled me but being the age I was I did not recognise what the feeling meant.

The major world events saw the hippy revolution shouting peace to all and Brazil had won the World Cup. Jason Tune entered another year at little Kimmy. I was going great guns at this time. Lady Bird books were being knocked off (read, in this case) at a fast rate. All my kings and queens could be recited at will and my crowning glory was to be one of the first in the class to be given a proper fountain pen to use. Promotion from book monitor to number one milk monitor was soon gained. I soon learnt a bit of capitalism here. One crate for me: the rest for the school. My first excursion into the black economy saw me flogging a bottle of milk to each of my adoring followers. They bought a bottle whether they wanted one or not. Who was arguing? Arguing? I was the main rooster. Black part or white in the playground, who was prepared to offer a challenge to the status quo? Always first in the dinner queue and a straight walk down the corridor. My swagger had more to do with watching old James Cagney movies at Grandma's house but it was enough for the tribal area of little Kimmy.

Chapter 2: Kimmy Kippers

Just like the army I began a recruitment drive. Not to serve my country but to form a like minded gang. I was never a bully, really, but even then I instinctively knew that a gang was a means of dispersing blame.

"There's them that do and them that thinks", said the Cap'n. Good advice. I will think and the rest can do it. I never had a particular rank name bestowed upon me but I was the number one as far as the rest went. I did have my second-in-command in the shape of Big Bob. My sub-lieutenant was a tough lad called Steffo. He was regarded as an 'up and coming' due to the fact that he had two pair of boxing gloves. Gentle persuasion from me meant that I had first call on borrowing them. The best pair of course.

Steffo's elder brother set up a make shift boxing ring in the Back Fields, a desolate area inhabited by mangy dogs, a few hangers on and us. Needless to say, it wasn't long before Steffo senior bit the dust after an introduction to yours faithfully.

Still, at least I learnt something from this brief bout of boxing. My opponents could lick dirt just as fast from boxing as from an unpaid bare-knuckle fight. The gang formed slowly and was based on a strict selection process. If someone was not providing a service or goods for general use (me first) then they were out. Like every group, we formulated our own set of rules and moral codes. I was first in the dinner queue, first pick for the daily footie match, first for the black one from the bag of sweets and total allegiance to the group. Dumb insolence was a matter of pride when confronted with someone in authority asking questions about us. Fear of me was the probable cause, but who is counting? This was just a game to me. On reflection I realise that my lack of comprehension as to the ramifications of my actions meant a straying from the good and proper. But maybe I did not listen to offered advice as well as I should have done. I was leader of the pack and it felt good. Odd times these. The Ties passing on their way to Big Kimmy (Kimberworth Comprehensive School) were always scrapping with each other. Gangs were formed left, right and centre in a blink of the eye. Unusual names were attached to the gangs to create an aura of power and supremacy.

Two, three, four scraps a day in the playground were commonplace. The girls were often worse than the boys. In an effort to ape the Big Kimmy gangs, our gang was officially named the Kimmy Kippers. Not exactly a name that would release fluid down the trouser leg of an opposing gang, but we thought it was hard and that was that. When Chez left Kimberworth Infants' School for advance studies at Meadowhall Road Junior School I took her place under the authoritarian gaze of Mrs. Fletcher. One look from her and hell would freeze over. Not to mention my inner strength and fast failing willpower. At least I did the stuff for her. My placement was a sort of introductory move to ease the pupil in with the form teacher. Surprisingly, she kept some of my schoolwork and at a later stage flourished it with great gusto under the noses of my younger brother and sister. In the run-up to the long awaited and long overdue (in my opinion) six weeks holiday I began to enjoy my schoolwork. My reading improved and so did my writing. My special pen was put to good use and I began to experience a new power: that of a swot.

Hurray, Hurray. The bell rang and the hordes piled out for six weeks of relaxing, chilling out and causing as much mayhem as we could. "Little bleeders", seemed to be the most oft quoted utterance. Closely followed by, "I know who you are and who your Father is". Our response of, "At least we know who our Father is," meant a quick dash to safety: The Back Field, of course. This was the badlands of Lower Kimberworth. We turned it into an adventure playground long before the concept of Centre Parks. The main attractions were the rope swing and ride of death (sliding down a short grassy bank, sat on a car bonnet). Stone throwing contests became a regular feature of the entertainment that was on offer. The target was usually some wannabe who had strayed onto the sacred sight in hopes of fun and acceptance. Climbing to the tree house, a cardboard box littered with left over dripping sandwiches, was always a must do activity. The highlight of the summer was the Holmes Hotel annual day trip to Skeggy (Skegness). On the coach, some adult would thrust a bag of food in our direction and our guardians handed over some spending money. What an experience. By ten O'clock everyone was skint. The penny arcades offering their chances to win a million pounds sucked up our meagre reserves like a desert having its first rain. By three O'clock we were all growling and thoughts of home and the fish and chips at the end of the journey were sending the stomach juices into ballet routines at a fast pace. Eight O'clock saw us outside the Meadowbank chippie with everyone claiming to have been on the first coach back. Tales of winning at least a fiver on the slot machines before eleven O'clock in the morning were changed to fifty pounds within minutes. If there was much more swearing down, Jesus would be visiting us. That, then, was my annual holiday. One day at the seaside. Good old days? UH!

Dave, my younger brother, once decided that he would go missing on the annual trip. This time we were at Costa Del Cleethorpes. Fish and chips were at four O'clock. on this trip and we all piled up to the allotted cafe. Dave was nowhere to be seen. There were five coaches so that meant five posses to look for him. At six thirty he was found on a policeman's lap, happy as a pig in muck, sucking an enormous lollypop without a care in the world. A few choice comments and the proverbial clip around the ear hole soon settled his hash. Not for the first time I wondered about him. He was too young to understand the concept of time and obligation. Dave had spent his time wandering about without a care in the world. More to come but the rain clouds of my future were yet to disturb my clear skies of the present. One day in the six weeks holiday a boy called Anthony from Upper

Kimberworth appeared. Within a few days he was a member of the gang and he was well liked. It was him who coined the nickname J instead of the full Monty of Jason. I thought that was well hard and distinguished me from the rest of the rank and file. Not for me the title of Field Marshall, but J. I liked that. J. And so it stuck. Mention J even now and some people still cower under their bed sheets or look decidedly guilty and give a 'I wish I wasn't here' look. Tony had a chopper bike with three gears. Naturally, J had first ride on the bike. The only trouble was my first turn lasted from dawn to dusk. Well, what is the point of being first if you can't be first? See. If truth were to be known he was effectively buying his way into the gang. Some people are easily bought and I am one of them. Only back in those days but definitely not now. My philosophies were coming along nicely. What's yours is mine and mine I keep. Soon, the holidays were over. These halcyon days were probably, in some ways, the most innocent of my life. Friendships were forgotten but soon to be replaced by the September rutting season's where the rankings were to be discussed and proved. My antlers were still the largest so it was only the minor positions that were up for grabs.

First day back, spic and span, ear holes washed and shoes shiny black. My adventures during the summer had finished and new challenges lay ahead. I strode into the playground, stood astride the black and white, arms folded. J was back. The troops touched their forelocks and offered their undying loyalty. This was thanks to my wonderful charm and the certain knowledge that I would level the disrespectful. My Lieutenants went about their business whilst I went about mine. This really was an uneventful year. The pecking order was sorted and my studies continued in the same vein as before. To tell the truth I was quietly proud of the fact that I was devouring my Ladybird books, especially the fairy stories. My Grandma enrolled me as a junior member of the library and my appetite for books increased. Never a word to my legions of fans, though. Who was I to destroy their myths? I was their fairy story albeit the nasty Godfather. My favourite books were about kings and queens. I soon stepped into the magic kingdoms that I read about and these flights of fancy took me roaming well beyond the backfield and the black and white parts of the playground.

All this reading changed my daydreams and I was no longer a pirate sailing with the Cap'n. My thoughts were of magical lands and daring dos. Life with Cap'n and his first mate Grandma continued along the same lines. A quick errand here and 'a take this' there. A couple of pence for sweets were still my goal and frequent visits to my parents' house. Open all hours was the theme of my parents and my growling stomach took full advantage of that. A quick raid of their pantry for much needed supplies, then back to the Cap'n's for a game of draughts or the card game Jazz.

One day, an Uncle of mine from my Mother's side appeared at the doorway with a Jack Russell pup. This was whilst I was having my monthly haircut or should I say monthly scalp at the hands of the Cap'n? "What thy doin wi that then?" was the utterance of Granddad. Uncle Ralph, more commonly known as 'Rice Pudding' due his total devotion to the stuff, explained that he had been down to check the bank account of the good people of Sheffield and he had found the Jack Russell pup. The pup had been abandoned in the sewerage works and looked very bedraggled and forlorn. Needless to say, a combination of "Can we have her?" every other minute and "Isn't she cute?" from Grandma lowered the resistance of Granddad. After the major exercise of cleaning her, grooming her and a baptism (Granddad dropped her in the bath) she was all ours. Trixie was my choice of name and it was duly bestowed upon her. I am not sure where the name came from but at the back of my mind I thought it was a character from a book. "One more mouth to feed", groaned the Cap'n. "We don't even get child allowance for other bugger". I smiled. Trixie was like a newborn kid. She slept in the bottom drawer and was winded every other minute. Trixie soon gained territorial rights to the area around the bottom drawer. No one went there unannounced. Subconsciously, I learnt from that. Thanks Trixie.

Around this time I started going to Sunday school. 'Owt for nowt' was the driving force. Regular attendance meant a bumper gift bag at Christmas and a rousing rendition of Onward Christian Soldiers brought nods of evangelic approval from the saved and a handful of sweets from the sweet jar at the end. The damned were saved and the damned were full of sweets. Odd, though, the louder and more fervent the singing the more sweets we had. 'Bloody bible bashers' was the scathing insult from the Ties in their mufti but who cared? We were eating sweets and they weren't. They were smoking, though. Perhaps Jesus did not save smokers.

So, I religiously attended Sunday school with my older sister Cheryl and the oldest sibling Marina. They called in for me before my weekly pilgrimage. I was duly inspected for neatness, cleanliness and for a clean handkerchief. I knew that my trial would soon be over, Lord, and a return to the house for the best Yorkshire puddings in Rotherham would follow. The Cap'n's Yorkshire puddings were renown throughout my kingdom. Some say, even to the lands beyond the top of Kimberworth. Onion gravy, roast potatoes, topside of beef and a generous dollop of 'Must I eat that green stuff?' were piled onto my plate. Treat of the week was, if truth was known, a slice of bread to mop up the gravy." Heaven". Yes, heaven was to be found on Sundays. What other day gave me sweets followed by piled high fodder within the space of one hour? Religion, that was for the pious. My stomach was the font of righteousness.

As soon as Trixie had finished off the beef bone I would dash off for another adventure with her in tow. She was my best mate and my trusted pal. She was my faithful companion and she was always pleased to see me. Dogs are consistent in their devotions and I responded in like to her. She was my special friend when no others were around.

The baby of the family was my youngest sister Samantha. There are four years and a month between us and in some respects she was more like a doll rather than a sister. I remember pushing her around in her pushchair for something to do rather than through sibling love. She had a kitten called Tibby but her cat and my dog never met. It was probably for the best, knowing the protective ferocity of Trixie. Samantha was closer to my brother Dave than me. This was entirely due to me living at my Grandparent's house. As she is the baby of the family I felt very protective towards her and still do. Sometimes, I used to read Samantha and Dave stories and on occasions make up stories to keep us all occupied. The made up story of the day was sometimes continued on another day. My readings gave me a land in which I roamed and Samantha and Dave were the recipients of my fertile imagination.

In the reality land where I roamed, the occupants of my kingdom were the challengers of my crown. Most of them more like court jesters rather than wandering knights. There were a few scraps going on amongst the lower ranks but no serious challenge came my way. As I have often thought, perceived power is achieved power. In my case it meant sitting on top of an opponent and pinning his shoulders to the deck. Breathing the question of 'Has tha had enough yet?' into the face of the unfortunate beneath me was the way a duel was sorted. Weight advantage and a touch of Jack Russell like ferocity made the rabble stand to one side in my presence. We were never sure about the pedigree of Trixie but my pedigree was not in doubt. The only serious challenge came from Big Bob. He stormed round to my house and accused me of taking his Tonka toy lorry without his consent. In the Wild West that would have been a hanging offence. But in lower Kimberworth that meant coats off and in the street for a head to head. Not for the first time Big Bob and I locked horns. Not for the last time Big Bob soon learnt that second was not good enough. My slight at being accused of being a thief was satisfied. Where I put the Tonka toy afterwards is still my secret but it doesn't do to admit anything when you are from lower Kimberworth. My reputation as being number one and also an honest friend was reinforced. Of course, we were best of mates the day after and peace descended once again upon my territory like the annual blessing at Christmas time. Christ is the saviour for those who fear God and I was the saviour of the rabble. If it wasn't me in charge they would have had Big Bob. He had no scruples, honour or morals. I had them in abundance. The fact that I metered out my standards in small doses was for the good of the troops. After all, too much too quick is not good. A mean, lean army is battle ready and my troops were certainly that with the rationing that I gave them. Big Bob was a greedy bugger and never saw the big picture. He was a bit of bully and the lower ranks were terrified of him. He would take all their sweets at one go. I would take only half of them. They thought that was a good deal. Fifty percent for them and the remainder paid to me. A bit like the tax system, they pay their whack and I don't whack them.

Chapter 3: The Unclassifieds

With a lump in my throat I left behind the Kimmy Infants and progressed into the first year of Meadowhall Road Junior School. After the obligatory line up and inspection in the yard I found myself paired off with Steffo but Big Bob was directed to another class. Parting is such a sweet sorrow but the lads from Meadowbank didn't cry.

To make up the third member of the Three Musketeers was Tony. Just as well that Big Bob was not with us. We needed teaching after all. I descended from number one in the Infants to a 'not sure' position in the Junior School. As I stood there surveying my new surroundings, a notable called Martin Black loped up to me and expressed his disapproval. The disapproval stemmed from the fact that I had sabotaged his homemade trolley. Trolleys were the toy of the moment. Everybody's trolley was faster, bigger, smarter looking or better designed than any other trolley, ever. He accused me of wrecking the brakes on his trolley. As it was morning break time and there was a full ten minutes to go before the bell we kicked off. Honours were even when the teachers parted us like the red sea in biblical times. By lunchtime, due to secret negotiations by the appointed unclassifieds, the time, the place and the wherefore was arranged. I dutifully turned up and off I went. Twenty sweaty minutes later with half the muck of lower Kimberworth stuck to us we stopped for a breather. "I'll get thee tonite", a panting M. Black snarled. "Four O'clock in the Back Field then", was my immediate reply. After all, always meet the enemy on your terms and on your patch. Thinking to myself that twenty minutes of sweaty endeavour was nineteen minutes too long I introduced my right fist to his over sized nose. A quick Ali shuffle meant the finish of Blackie. I could feel the elevation up the ranks happening again. "Cor, did you see that?" said one of the bespectacled pant wetters. From one punch thrown it developed into a massacre with no one quite dead. Who was I to tell the truth? Better the myth than reality. The more who talked about it the more my reputation was enhanced. Global warfare stood at a five foot high. With an attempted swaying of the hips I strolled into Junior School the next day. "Hi J", came from every corner of the playground. Some of the junior four boys grunted an 'Ah Reight'. My only slight reservation was when an older mate of Blackies would come round for the give back or return as we used to say.

My schoolwork was going at a good rate and I would often receive a gold or silver star for my efforts. Before I knew it Christmas was upon us again. This time I knew for sure that Father Christmas was not real. Little did I know it but the last vestige of innocence had gone. No more fairy stories, no more make believe, just hard reality. Due to watching and fantasising about the ancient gladiators (no difference there then ... considering what was to come) led my Father to buy me some plastic replica amour. I duly turn up at school in the New Year resplendent in my amour announcing my name as Julius J. The first task was to receive the oath of the gladiators (to me naturally) and in the absence of a ferocious lion we went off to ambush Big Bob. He was trying to recruit a gang behind our backs but in the event even Spartacus would not have had much luck. Without too much trouble, and thanks to my protective apparel, Big Bob was once again regulated to foot servant status. I was unbeatable with my amour on. Until of course the rulers of the school i.e. the teachers suggested that I took off my 'silly outfit'. I have had the last laugh because even today people relate the story of legionnaire Julius J.

That year the current cup holders, Leeds United, were back at Wembley and my life long support for the team was set. My Father took me to the nearest department store and bought Dave and me a Leeds United replica shirt. I felt proud as a peacock. "Dus thy 'ave a bath in that shirt, Tuney?" was one of the mildest comments offered to me at the time. A reply of "At least I have a bath" usually meant a quick exit. An early obsession with the Leeds player Peter Lorimer meant that my hair became longer and more unkempt. My interest in playing football developed and I even joined the Salvation Army in order to play for a team. I needed salvation but the Sally Army was the last place to find it. Every available minute was being spent on playing football. All over the field was my favourite position. The football became such a time filler that little time was being spent on the ranking of J. Tune. Friendships were being formed at a fast rate and the basis of life long friends stemmed from the football matches. Tactics formed on the playing fields of Eton had nothing on us.

As spring blew into Lower Kimberworth the days were growing longer and more time was being devoted to playing out. Marbles soon became the second favourite passion of the five-foot populace. The major game was played in the now demolished old school arches. A popular myth was that the place was visited by a ghost at precisely whatever time I said it was. At the sound of my cry that the 'Green Lady' was here meant a huge rush to the available exits. The over excitable deluded believers left behind many of their marbles including 'queens and pearlies'. So one night I played my game and off went the 'scaredy cats'. As I was bending down to pick up my spoils I came face to face with the quietest kid in school known as Mick the Bomb. Easy meat, thought I, and I told him what to do with himself. Without further ado he went for it. He was a total underestimation on my part. It was one of the hardest fights I had that year. On reflection it was probably the hardest fight of any year. For the first time I sensed the feeling of inadequacy. From somewhere within me came the will to succeed and I finally managed to put him to rest. Phew! There were more bouts to come with him but the psychological advantage of winning was always with me. Never underestimate anybody was one of my mottos but only to me. Let the ranks think differently. What they did not know did not matter. If they did know it would only have traumatised them so perhaps I did them a favour by ensuring that their safe environment and place in life was without question. A smile took over before I went to sleep that night. No dreams though.

Mind you, no bragging about that particular fight the next day. I did not want to fight him seven days per week. One defeat in a thousand would not go down well with the lower ranks.

The buzz about the Olympics was still doing the rounds and the teachers used it as examples of achievement and interest. I recall doing a project on Mary Peters and I found myself totally immersed in the work. Any adverse comment from any of the contenders was met with a sideways glance. Sometimes a timely crack on the head was not always necessary. I was beginning to learn that perceived power means assumed power.

My studies meant a lot to me and I enjoyed collating the information that I needed. In a strange way, my relentless questions to my family brought me closer to the adult versions of the Tunes. As a Tune, albeit a junior type, my place and role was intrinsically defined within the family culture but my Mary Peters project opened channels of communication previously denied me. Suddenly, I was involved in discussions and members of my family began to ask me on a daily basis how my work was coming along. Grunts and snarls on a frequent basis gave way to sentences and verbal communication. Odd to think that at one time I was almost monosyllabic but this opening of downwards respect and interest in my direction led me to realise that I could talk and talk well. In the book 'A Christmas Carol' by Dickens there is a line that says, "If any man knew how to keep Christmas well it was Scrooge". It has often been said of me since the Mary Peters project that if any man can talk well it is certainly Tune.

Of course the new ace communicator still reverted to other methods of giving out messages, especially to a nasty smell known by the nickname of Meany Deanie. This lad began to pick off one or two of the more notable members of the gang. Even Steffo was taken out. He lost a little too easily for my liking. Not that I was bothered but I expected more from Steffo. One day, someone jokingly said to me that it would be my turn soon. I reminded this lower rank that he was not even supposed to talk to me but through one of my Lieutenants. Having been said, however, it was to prove difficult to avoid. Enough said. The fight coordinators were summoned and two of the gang were sent off to arrange the where, the when and the engagement rules. There were no rules but tradition had to be observed. To my amazement the fight was arranged in an alternative venue. Across the main road of the estate, would you believe? Thus was the importance of this fixture. On the appointed day, there were lookouts posted at every corner to watch out for passing elders, parents or the enemy (police). No kicking, no joining, no pulling hair and definitely no scratching, intoned the referee. Whilst this self-elevated glory seeker was doing his pre fight warm up I landed the first blow. Or should I say the last blow? He was blown out quicker than Marilyn Monroe's candle. The watchers-on were in some part amazed and in some parts disappointed that J. Tune was still standing. Another notch on the Lonsdale, or should I say, the Lower Kimberworth belt?

Unbeknown to me Meany Deanie's Mum and my Mother were close gossips and even closer tea swilling partners. When we thought that news of our altercation across the road had reached their ears, the feud was quickly dissolved. Instead, we became good friends and I often went round to his house at night to play monopoly or better still with his marble collection. Massive collection, that was. Far too mean a person to ever take it to school. The food at Deanie's house was legendary and that suited me fine. It was bangers and mash on a good day or mash and bangers on a poor day. Sundays, there was gravy as well. Forks were optional. Due to the defeat of Steffo, Meany Deanie joined the gang and he took over Steffo's duties. No fixed roster, just walking about with the air of a gang member, complete with the imitation J. Tune swagger.

To the family's great joy, and feeling of one up man ship, my Father bought a Jaguar car. This purchase of the next family vehicle was more a result of relocated scrap than the wages of honest endeavour. Working on the rule if it's not bolted down it is fair game many purchases were made that defied the taxman's assessments. Many considered him a colourful character but some were distinctly uncomfortable when near him. J. Tune might have been the boy of the family but my Father was certainly the Daddy of the town. There was a rumour that he used to charge a toll for people just to pass through the town centre. Complete nonsense but every bit helps when creating a living myth. His job was very physical and so was he. Cosmetic surgeons have nothing on his ability to rearrange the looks of people. It was said that he was a bit of a ladies man but no proof fell my way. General gossip forged many an unproven statement but they always follow a reputation. One thing about my Father that was true was his muscular physique. Hard work and regular sessions on the weights kept him in fighting trim. As he wasn't a boxer it would be more accurate to say that he kept himself in fine knuckling condition. He introduced himself to many would be's and made sure that they ended up as never could be's.

He was at his peak and I still had a fair way to go. The king was not even a prince yet but I was an integral part of the Tune dynasty. The name Tune was revered but I was pursuing my own agenda of being known as J. My title was J and I was intent on making the junior inhabitants of the Kimberworth area sit up and take notice. One or two adults were sending a few questioning glances in my direction when I passed and hands were beginning to cover mouths as softly spoken words were muttered to one another. Not through respect. I suspect that what they were really saying was "Little so and so", but the family name and reputation restricted their desires to speak out loud. Pride. What was this new found feeling? It was a strange emotion. Unrecognised but welcoming. Whilst not being entirely sure about the full significance of pride, and its full impact, it rested well with me. I instinctively knew that it was something that I should never lose. Over the years this pride of mine was to prove to be the mainstay of my life and sometimes the central pillar onto which to hang to when things were at their lowest.

However, that was for the future and I had the small matter of keeping my kingdom in check. Daily sorties to discourage insurrection by the lower ranks and a few snarls here and there at the dogs of war of the inner sanctum of the gang were my basic ploys. As a Junior School urchin, I could not rationalise my feelings or thoughts. Potential repercussions of my actions were not my thinking or consideration. I just went out and did what I did best. That was, the keeping of order of the unclassifieds and the quelling of any possible insurrection. What that meant exactly I did not know but my gut instincts were to defend my right to rule and to rule totally. I was just a kid. But what a kid, said some.

End of another school year and all thoughts were focussed on the six weeks school holidays. This was a time to play, to forge friendships and a time to cause mayhem. Not surprisingly, I helped my Grandparent's quite a lot during the holidays. Eight bells would find the Cap'n and me off to the shops for the daily victuals. Inevitably, a couple of bottles of brown stout (for medicinal purposes) would be included. Most mornings I would escort my Grandma down to the town centre for meat and fresh bread. This seemed to be the way of it for many kids and I would see many of my ranks out and about. Most afternoons there would be a gathering of the clans, or to be more precise, those that counted. Football, tree climbing and the eating of dripping sandwiches filled our days. Not that I was noticing, but I was growing again. Upwards and outwards to such an extent that one night, straight after tea, there was a meeting of all concerned on the quarter deck. The Cap'n, with his dog by his side, stood up to speak. "Nah den, listen you lot", he intoned. "Bleeding little sod 'ere has been eating me out of house and harbour and he's got too big for his britches". So, the very next day, after the war council had agreed on a price, I went for my first grown up long trousers. With much grumbling and lots of "SHHH, don't swear in here", the Cap'n and his faithful first mate finally, to the shopkeeper's relief, poured me into a pair of long trousers. My, it felt strange, especially the itching feeling on tender legs. The journey home was a trial in its own right. Never have I been given so much advice on what to do and what not to do and what would happen if I did do it. I had not so much been bought a pair of trousers but a robe of the finest most expensive silk. Later, when I was standing next to my friends, I felt as if I was more grown up than them. Of course, there was some friendly banter from my mates and, naturally, there was some not so friendly retaliation from yours truly. The days passed and all too soon the clarion call back to school sounded. A collective sigh was heard round the leafy suburbs of Lower Kimberworth as the unwilling trudged towards the penal colony of the Junior School. For once, and not the last time as it turned out, I grudgingly went off to school on a sharp but windy day in early September.

The first major project attempted by the rabble, was one on the meaning of the autumn season. Collecting leafs was good fun as it meant time out of the classroom. Gluing the leaves and the rest of the collectables proved to be a nightmare as the Captain's dire warnings rang around my head. Long trousers. A curse and a blessing at the same time. The long trousers also had the side effect of confusing the Cap'n's dog, Trixie. She started to follow me every time I went off to school. She must have thought that I was the Cap'n on one of his jaunts. One day, she followed me out of the house and all the way to school. The first I knew of it was when I was going into my classroom. Despite whispering commands through my clenched teeth to order her home she trotted into the classroom. I was beside myself but the rank and file thought it was a hoot. "Mr. Smith is here", came the cry from the appointed lookout and I dashed to my seat with Trixie at my feet. It was not that long before Mr. Smith spotted Trixie underneath the desk. I suppose the give away was the giggling of the troops and the whimpers of Trixie. He came storming round to my desk and wagged a finger in the direction of Trixie whilst telling me in no uncertain terms the errors of my ways. During the explanation that this was a classroom and not a dog kennel, Trixie decided to respond to the conversation by the inappropriate action of nipping the wagging finger. The last I remember of the event was the howls of laughter from the enlisted and the howls of anguish from the suited one. The last comment by one unknown, "If Tuney does not get them, the dog will", finished the affair. My journey back to school was not one I wanted to do. This story still does the rounds and has long descended into the folklore of Lower Kimberworth.

The teacher, Mr. Smith, due no doubt to his Christian beliefs, did not hold the incident against me. Rather, he took an unexpected shine to me. On a few occasions he took me to the Pentecostal Church for a rendering of guitars, tambourines and out of tune singing. Who cared? Certainly not me. There was great fodder to be had in the kitchen area and rations were rations as far as I was concerned. The highlight of the early evening singsong was a liberal amount of proper fizzy pop. Almost a rare thing on the estate. 'Now't wrong wiv watter' was the usual excuse offered for not buying the childhood nectar. A calling to the higher levels of Christian understanding was beyond me but these excursions to the oasis of truth and enlightenment, at least instilled in me a sense of respect for the older members of society, as and when they deserved it. I have always maintained a polite mode of behaviour and a respect for other people's property. A respect that stretches to the one unshakable truth: if it belongs to someone I like, then it is theirs. Otherwise!

Another thing that Mr. Smith did was to transport me and a Tune selected gang consisting of Steffo and the two best-looking girls at the time to a park on the other side of Sheffield. Strange land this was. People were sitting on rugs and kids eating ice cream as if wartime rationing was still in existence. Nice days though. What could be better than a walk in the park with two beautiful girls? Pity I did not know quite what to do with them. Just as well. The good citizens of inner Abbeydale would have choked over their morning cup of tea at the vicarage. A good man was Mr. Smith. In some ways he was responsible for a calm and uneventful year regarding the macho display of brawn and burgeoning muscle. In school I developed a love for sums and number work. As the ranks did not gain much success in this aspect of education, I used it as a weapon against them. What you can't always fight, then out think. Silver awards were not enough and I would make every effort to obtain a rare and much deserved gold award. My football skills were improving and I began to play whenever I could. Although I have always wrote with my right hand I would favour my left foot when playing football. Bit by bit my strength increased in my shooting and kicking a football. It was not only the football that I kicked. During one match I mistimed my tackle and follow through and kicked a different type of ball. The resulting screams from the poser were enough to turn the stomachs of the most hardened bystander. Norman Hunter of Leeds United was called 'Bite your legs Hunter'. I became known, for a short while, as 'kick your knackers off Tuney". Nothing new there then?

This year was in some ways the most uneventful year of my primary and secondary schooling. The academic year ended with a huge surprise to all us urchins of Lower Kimberworth land. It was time for my first ever school trip. A "grand day out" had nothing on this charabanc trip. I was at school before the caretaker's cat had caught its first mouse such was my excitement. The sight of so many clean knees was in itself a sight to behold. My long trousers, now carefully turned up in the style of the 'Ties', were as sharp as the village gossips tongue. In my hand was a bag of fodder that could have fed the class and half the rats on the beach at the canal lock. The noise of the excited chatter reached a crescendo when the cry of 'It's here' went up. As soon as the coach stopped the scrum for the back seated started. When the dust of the troops had settled I decided to introduce myself to the bespectacled unclassifieds occupying what was to me my rightful place. With one click of my fingers the fawning pawns scattered in a mixture of fear and pride at having made the back seat for at least two minutes. So I settled in the prime seat with a girl on each arm for company and a nominated batman serving me dolly mixtures at my behest. The engine grumbled to life and with a roar from the now hyper juveniles, matched only by the crowd at Wembley on Leeds United's greatest day, the coach set off on its epic journey to unknown lands and strange people. The coach stopped at Conisbrough Castle, near Doncaster. We did not know that we had gone about 15 miles. Our stomachs were aching with the flood of sweets and sandwiches that were washed down with copious amounts of pop. During the journey I tried vainly to swap my dripping sandwiches for something more appealing. No deal. Even the unclassifieds declined my generous offer. I let it pass. Our day consisted of mock Norman and Tudor battles. Sometimes I rewrote history judging by the number of troops who picked up, battlefield injuries representing the historical winners. Memories flooded back when one wise cracking teacher said, "Tuney, where's tha armour?" Funny bugger! I could not quite understand sarcasm but I knew that I had been outsmarted somehow by some means but only temporarily.

The only blot on the day was when 'there is always one' could not hold his bowels until the end of the return journey. He was, unfortunately, sat a couple of seats up from me. Phew! I soon scampered down the coach to escape the miniature Blackburn Meadows erupting with a venomous force behind me. Or should I say him? For what seems to be forever he is still referred to as 'Honies' (as in sweet as Honies).

Later that year I was allowed to go collecting bonfire wood. This was a big event for me as usually it was the 'Ties' who carried out this admired task. First job was to acquire a settee and chair for guard duties. Every bommie (bonfire) had its selected legionnaires to guard against infiltrators and skanks. The bommie grew and grew through a combination of polite requests and an active relocation programme. That meant of course that our bommie was more susceptible to raiding parties. Everyone was nominated for night duties. A place was reserved on the settee along with a campfire to keep you warm. One night, a certain Tie by the name of Lofty came along to remove our ill-gotten gains. As he was following a personal 'help your self system' one of our gang knocked the centre pole straight on the top of Lofty's head. He just managed to keep enough sense to pick him self up and run. In some ways this event was a shock to me. Until then I had always settled my affairs with my fists. To see a weapon being used was out of context to what I was about. The Cap'n always used to say that the one who pushed the centre pole was a sly one. He never allowed him into the house. As things turned out the Cap'n was proved to be one hundred percent right.

On the lead up to bonfire night I became quite the entrepreneur. I used the Cap'n's favourite hatchet to make bundles of firewood for the coal fires. There were plenty of customers for my under priced bundles and the profits were used for buying yet more fireworks and especially toffee apples. 'Guy Fawking' took place outside the Meadowbank Hotel with my sisters for an hour or two. There was never a question of whose patch it was. It was ours, full stop. One night, just as we were about to cash in, a boy called Paddy turned up. He started to pull our Guy Fawkes apart and demanding the money. As this boy was three years older than me I stood back at first. When he laid hands on Marina I exploded. To everyone's surprise I soon ended up on the top of him and gave him my personal brand of fire works. First, a Roman Candle, followed by a blow that made his eyes go round faster than the Catherine Wheel finished him off for good. The assembled crowd, mostly blokes who were leaving the pub, gave me a generous round of applause. It was not the victory that tasted sweet. It was the acknowledgement from the crowd.

My reputation soared especially as Paddy came from an area known as the Bottom Field. The Bottom Field Mob were regarded as not quite being on the map, so any sorting out of one of their crowd was greeted with great glee. The talk back at school the following week was how Tuney had vanquished the foe, especially one that was three years older.

For me it was business as usual. Big deal. So what? I was the man, or in this case the boy. What I did with Paddy seemed to me to be my destiny. It was what I did. No question. No doubts. The troops and the unclassifieds fell over themselves in the re-telling of the 'Paddy' saga. It went from the truth to a savage beating that left him in hospital. The rumour control board were having a field day. I did nothing to discourage such adulation. What that meant exactly I did not know but it made me feel taller and more important. Not so much egoistical but more the need to be number one.

I sat back and did my schoolwork and did the things that kids normally do. Girlfriends, football and eating sweets were the main agenda. The rumour mill continued and I carried on in my own way. School was still proving to be a challenge to me. It was one that I relished, if truth be told. If someone called me a swot they would have been regulated to an unclassified state in double quick time. I enjoyed my schoolwork to such an extent that I had a buzz every time I produced good work. A red 'Well done' from the teacher was hidden from view but it meant a lot to me on a personal level. The other school challenge to me was for me to play in the school 'A' side. Unfortunately, only the last year group at school was allowed to play in the 'A' team and I had to settle for the 'B' team for one year. Despite my best efforts, even I could not defeat officialdom in the disguise of the teachers. I made up for my disappointments by continually playing football at night or at the weekends with older kids. Football was becoming my passion and way of life. Every scrap of information about my beloved Leeds United was devoured and repeated at great length. Also, at this time, I managed to achieve my swimming competence certificate. No great deal but at least it prevented my parents from going on at me about swimming in the local canal. They thought I could swim to London and back but it was more like spitting distance with lots of swallowed water. Although I loved my swimming lessons I really did hate the rigmarole at the swimming baths. As a Lower Kimberworth freebie I was regarded as a carrier of every known foot disease to mankind. All the kids from my end of town went through the same rigorous inspection before the lesson started. Good job it was swimming and not underwear modelling. The embarrassment of being sent back into the changing rooms for another scrub or clean down was at times too much to bear. Even we likely lads had our pride and emotions. Still, the Tune won through and the certificate was mine.

Christmas time heralded my propulsion to a leading role in the annual nativity play at school. My role was that as one of the three kings. In my view there was only one king but I let it pass. Two unclassifieds made up the numbers. My role was at the forefront again. The play went well and I received quite a lot of praise for my involvement. Odd come to think about it. I have always flirted with religion and some of religion has, in some ways, flirted with me. Not so much the full-blown church service but more the philosophical aspects of religion have appealed to me. Straight after the nativity play we piled into my classroom for the Christmas party. Instead of the usual offering of two slightly dried dripping sandwiches I arrived at school with a chocolate cake and crisps. Thanks mainly to the Cap'n's first mate. The party was in full swing when a particularly nasty brand of human rejection entered the room. Was it a boy or was it girl? A Scottish lump, that resembled an overgrown Satsuma on a bad day more than a person. This was the notorious newcomer from Edinburgh called Lesley. Even her/his name was in doubt let alone his/her sexuality. Les, and there were rumours to that effect, came into the room and announced in her broad Scottish accent, "Uuuse yuus lukin at, jimmy". I could not work out if it was an insult or not due to the fact that I could not understand her/him. What I did understand was the fact that she had offered me out. Me! Was this a Christmas cracker joke gone wrong? No, she meant business. Four O'clock she said. Hang on; thought I that is football time. So, without further ado, I gave her a Christmas present that was not on her Father Christmas wish list. It was not gift-wrapped but it was definitely a present that I wanted to give her. This was to be the first and most definitely the last girl that I ever had a fight with. All I know is that my stock with the rest of the girls went sky high. They were terrified of her and now I was the protector of all fair damsels in distress. My early training with my armour certainly paid dividends. In the aftermath of this exchange I pointed out to her that there was only one Meadowbank and it was in Rotherham and not Scotland. The girl Lesley spent the next few years snarling and spitting but, as with the way of it, she eventually became a pal.

One night, I called into my parents place for a bit of supper. As it turned out, they were out for the evening and a girl was babysitting David and Samantha. They were asleep and she was sitting on the settee. She looked at me and asked me if I wanted to go upstairs to play 'doctors and nurses'. Yeah, I was game for that. So up the stairs we went. By the time she had my long trousers down and wrapped her warm hands round my functional bit I began to realise that she was playing a different game to me. Not knowing the rules I just stood there whilst my symbol of maleness changed size and feeling. All I knew was that something enjoyable was happening but I hadn't a clue what to do about it. My hesitation was spared when Samantha shouted for her. I hastily zipped up and legged it as fast as I could to the Cap'n's

berth. To my surprise I was red as a beetroot and sweating like the proverbial. My first sexual experience was a disaster in terms of uninformed innocence. I resolved there and then that I would find out as much as I could about the mysteries of sex and find out myself what to do and more importantly how to do it. There were to be more fumblings of a farcical nature before I was the Don Juan of El Rotherham.

The highlight of the academic year was the winning of the 'B' team all Rotherham schools knockout soccer cup. Knockout was not what the organisers had in mind when we applied our version of knockout during matches. Due to the fact that my school could not afford proper football nets, we tended to play all our matches away. Our tactics were quite simple. Big Bob ambled over to the other side's biggest lad and he spelled out in detail what the consequences would be if our side lost. The sight of yours truly and Steffo entering the arena was usually the last straw for the hapless opponents. As the appointed Captain of the team I had the honour of receiving the cup in a special school assembly. This was probably the proudest moment of my Junior School days and I remember the event with clarity and a huge sense of achievement.

This feeling of euphoria lasted well through the six weeks holidays and all too soon the call to morning lessons resounded round the district. My return to Meadowhall School was with the rank of commander. Of course, there were those who wished to threaten the rightful chain of command and, of course, it was mainly the usual suspects.

Mick the Bomb was an ugly looking specimen with jagged teeth and the breath to go. This ambitious likely lad had, unbeknown to many, been training furiously through the summer months at martial arts. Remember, this was the time of Kung Fu and Bruce Lee wannabees. He was the silent but deadly type and he was always on the look out for a chance to try his luck. A second Dan, at a pub called the Miners Arms on Meadowbank Road, trained him. The sort of place where someone could buy whatever they wanted before it was acquired for sale. It resembled an early Argos without V.A.T. The trouble with Mick the Bomb was that going 'ooh aah' at a punch bag was not the same as going full tilt with J. Tune. He kicked off in the Patio area between our respective classrooms. As it was break time the rent a crowd turned up baying for blood and a few tears as well. He went into the stance of the crouching tiger and he soon ended up in the stance of the sprawled dormouse. Just like the saying goes: It's no use fastening wings to a dead duck. It's still a dead duck. The assembled audience shouted their exultations but to me it was a case of one comes and another goes. Unfortunately, the noise attracted the attention of the warders and we were hauled off to the head teacher's office. I stood there expecting the usual 'Don't be naughty boys routine' when to my total shock he reached for his cane on the top of his cupboard and swished the rod with the expertise of a Musketeer. It hurt. Not that I let on. Pride is pride after all. The wails of Mick the Bomb were at once disgraceful and wimpish.

With the words of the head teacher ringing in my ears I went back to my class with the unsaid promise that I would try my best with my work. No one was foolish enough to criticise me so I launched myself into my class work with fervour. Once I had discovered what creative writing was all about, my imagination knew no bounds. Thoughts and ideas flowed from the school biro of yours truly and five or six pages were not uncommon. Some of the newly released from their Mother's aprons strings could not even spell their name. A few visits to different museums further triggered my imagination and thirst for knowledge. York railway museum kept me going for weeks on end. Not so much the Flying Scotsman but the Flying Tune. One day, we went to the main museum in York. The highlight of that visit was to lie on the iron bed that was in the alleged cell that Dick Turpin occupied. This was known as the condemned cell. Why it felt at home I couldn't say, funny that.

Whilst I was bashing out yet another magnificent tome two girls appeared at the side of me. They were giggling in the way that they do. These two intermediaries produced the note that meant everything. For a couple of weeks I had been processing the bush telegraph that I fancied the blonde bombshell known as Tilly. The deal was made with Steffo tagging along to make up the numbers with Tilly's mate, Sandy. As befitting the good time lads we took them swimming to the canal. Not a bad move really. At least we did not have the pre-swimming baths inspection. In order to impress the women or girls the macho man stood on the swing bridge and dived in to the canal with the sound of applause ringing in his ears. Of course, J.Tune being J.Tune had to dive in from the top girder. With gasps and ooohs going round like a verbal Mexican wave I smiled at the crowd and dived in. Tilly loved me forever after that. On the way home my hand slipped into her hand. At the corner before her house I kissed her. Lovely. I kissed her again. At that moment I knew that women were to be a part of me like eating, breathing and going to sleep. Romance was to be an acquired thing but in those far flung days of yesterday romance meant calling the girlfriend bird and kissing whilst chewing gum. Next day, the first of many taunts were heard on the battlefield, sorry, the playground. Tuney is now a soft one. Secretly I felt pleased and a bit more grown up.

This romance lasted a whole three weeks before the dramatic break up. Her parents found out about the romance and she was immediately banned from seeing a Lower Kimberworth lad. I knew something was wrong with this decision but I did not understand in those days. Prejudice never reared its head in the Lower Kimberworth Precinct so I could not see what the fuss was all about. No one said anything to me and I said not a word to anyone. There were no problem pages to write to at that time so problems were kept in house.

My frustrations were released in the football matches. Suddenly, the team became the most important thing in my life. After Tony's Father bought the school some football nets, the school started to play more matches at home. After a while, I started to travel with the Rotherham under 11's football team. That year we had a fabulous cup run. In one memorable match we played in deep snow at Ilkeston and won 6-0. Eventually, we reached the final and lost narrowly after extra time to Sheffield Boys.

Just before festive holidays of the last year at Junior School, Big Bob decided to have another tilt at the windmill. As he could not play in the football team he started to associate with a group of Ties led by Gasping Gaz, the sly one who the Cap'n had warned against. Big Bob fired the bullets that Gasping Gaz gave him. The target was me. At the end of my road were some fabricated garages and it was here that a gang of Ties caught up with me. Out of one of the empty garages strolled Big Bob. He started to swear at me and offered me out. Bolstered by the presence of his so-called mates he thought that this was the opportunity to have a go. Third time lucky or so he thought. Third time it was. He hit the ground. I put my parka back on and as my back was turned he leapt on me. Kick off time again. Second half. Drawing nil-nil with ten minutes to go, a right hand cross followed by a firm head ended all hopes of a revival by the minnow. 3-0. At this point, the realisation that his mates were still there hit me. For once, the odds were stacked against me. The only course of action I could think off was to snarl in their general direction and slowly wander off. There were lots of chants and name calling but sometimes discretion is the better part of not having your head kicked in. My relationship with Big Bob was definitely a none starter. I hardly spoke to him until the following September when I made my grand entrance to the 'Land of the Ties'.

Chapter 4: Slag Bin... Home of Northern Soul

My entrepreneurial skills developed during the school year and I cornered the lucrative crisp market at break times. Even though the teachers knew what I was doing, due to my newly acquired status as teacher's pet I was allowed to continue my activities. I sold crisps, buns and other eatables. The profits paid for my first pair of high waisters. These were the most fashionable trousers at the time and they were the type of thing that followers of Northern Soul wore. Lunchtimes saw my negotiation skills at their finest. By the time I had finished I had more on my food plate than I should have. Who is complaining? A growl is a growl and boy was I growling. My appetite was ferocious and I made sure that it was kept in check.

For some reason, chess seemed to be the intellectual pursuit amongst the boffs and those with more than half a brain cell. Naturally, I joined in. Being a top set lad and the teachers' pet I welcomed the invitation to attend the chess club. The leading protagonist at chess was an odd-bod by the name of Henry John, John being the American for something else and I sometimes wonder how right they are. Boy was he odd. He was however a competent chess player and remained unbeaten for most of the time that he was in Junior School. That was until I decided that this was a challenge that I could not turn down. After school tuition, secret lessons and mentorship by members of my family who could play put me into the position of challenger for the chess crown. My pre-match Mohammed Ali hype up meant that I had to play him fair and square and not put the frighteners on him. In waded the unclassifieds who thought that they could smell a defeat of yours truly with no cost to themselves. All week the talk on the streets, or should I say playground, was the imminent defeat of the Tune. To tell the truth a certain doubt crossed my mind. Losing a battle was one thing; to lose a mental challenge was another thing. Still, the time came and I sat down opposite the odd-bod. Shake hands, said the teacher. Not on your life, thought I. I was not sure if oddness was physically transmitted. The room was full of a whispering eager crowd. A cough was greeted with stern looks and offers of punching the coughers' lights out. Odd-bod moved a pawn. A white pawn. The reigning champion was always white. The first drop of sweat dribbled down my back. What was this? My palms were sticky. With a nervous hand I countered his opening move. I sat back with a smile on my face. Not that I was feeling confident but more a reaction to my nerves. When the gasp of surprise, intrigue and what the hell was that all about went up, odd-bod looked distinctly gone. He was the one who was nervous and trembling. Let the others worry about you came to mind. Where that came from I was not sure but it was a familiar saying to me.

Twenty-two minutes later I moved my king's rook and pronounced check mate. Odd-bod looked even odder. Most of the crowd could not understand that I had won or how. All that the unclassifieds knew was that yet another opportunity to see the Tune fall from grace had passed them by. Suckers. Tune, the chess king. I let humility sweep over me. Only for a second though. Odd-bod spoilt my moment of triumph by crying his eyes out. Within a second I had gone from the King to the executioner. Another war won on a different battlefield. Yippee.

Easter holidays had arrived. This meant chocolate Easter eggs and free time. What more does a boy need for himself? What more? A haircut. Off I was dragged to barber John at the top of the lane. My Father sat me in the chair and told barber John to give me a Northern Soul haircut. Was I pleased! The full works. Shampoo for starters followed with all the smellies. Finally, after the feathering and snipping and shaving was the blow wave back. By this stage barber John was getting quite excited. I was becoming more nervous. He was often referred to as the limp wrist barber. Being quite the innocent shy boy that I was I had no idea what being limp wrist entailed. Only that it did entail tail. Now I understand why my Father accompanied me to the den of opportunity. I cannot bring myself to give him his correct title. My years have proved to be totally against that side of human activity. I strutted around for days with my new hairstyle.

My oldest sister Marina decided that it was time for me to learn how to soul dance. Her current boyfriend of the time was a D.J. in his spare time and he volunteered to bring along some records and teach me some moves. For such a cumbersome uncoordinated youth I took to soul dancing like a duck to water. Smooth on the surface and paddling furiously underneath. This led me to going to a youth club on a Thursday night that played Northern Soul stuff. Although I was probably too young to go I was regarded as cool and in I went. The place was commonly known as the Slag Bin. Judging by the amount of girls having a colloquial bin ender outside, no wonder it had the name. I, of course, being a quiet shy boy never indulged. I preferred to think of it as a serious romance lasting all of ten minutes. If she did not have bad breath it stretched to fifteen minutes. Bad breath resurrected itself years later and that is why I mention it now.

My dancing came on leaps and bounds or should I say backdrops and splits? Soul Spins King was my early Slag Bin nickname before J took over. My kingdom was taking longer to conquer than I thought but I was getting there.

One day the Cap'n demanded my immediate and undivided attention to a small detail outside the house. A fence had blown over and he was repairing it. Hold it still whilst I hit it, he said. I thought he meant the nail. He thought he meant the nail. The nail in question was the nail on my now squashed finger. I became aware of the fallibility of my Grandparent's and that they were beginning to grow old. The Cap'n's eyesight wasn't all it should have been and he had forgotten to put his glasses on. He never forgot again. My glasses had hit the bottom of the outside bin weeks before. No longer did I carry the burden of the squint or the hushed barbed comment of Clarence.

My last term at Junior School was mostly filled up with revision for the final end of term exams. These exams were supposed to determine what set we went into when we reached the big school. I read all the junior encyclopaedias and revised my guzzintas with a vengeance. (Two goes into four twice). Eventually the exam days arrived. The dining hall was cleared and desks arranged in none copying order. Armed with sharpened pencils, a new pen and brimming with confidence, I thought to myself: bring it on. Bring it on they did but I was up for the challenge. Another battle won. Although it was to be a while before the results were announced, I knew from my after match discussions that I had done more than all right. I was proved to be right.

Just before the end of term, a group of Ties descended on the school banking. Ciggies lit and much swearing was the order of the day. Naturally, I wandered out to determine what the visit was for. One of the Ties told me that a kid from another feeder school was looking for me and wanted to kick my head in. This was the first time that I had encountered professional bullet providers. They were talking up a fight for their entertainment when they returned to school in the autumn term. Due to the fact that for quite a while I had not been in with anybody, I was distinctly disturbed by this piece of information. I was expecting to go to the big school and swan along in my own way when suddenly I had a challenge without even seeing the guy. No comment was my way of reacting to the wind up and I left them as soon as I could. When I saw my Father that same evening I told him about the visit. He suggested that it was about time that I joined his body building gym that he ran in the Royal George pub at Meadowbank.

I trained three times per week throughout the summer holidays usually with my brother Dave. My Father became my personal coach but just because I was eleven and his Son did not mean that he spared the tongue lashes and ridicule. He was a powerful guy and a known figure in the town. Although I did not realise it, my physique began to change. My power increased, as did the size of most bits of me. 'He'll knacker his joints up', was the grumpy remark of the Cap'n. I now realise that my Father suspected that I was in for a turbulent time at the big school and this was his way of preparing me for the taking of Kimberworth Comprehensive School.

Chapter 5: Precinct Kimmy

Monday morning, bright and early, I surveyed my new kingdom. I joined the milling throng that was swirling around at the top of the drive that the teachers used to access the school. Tall and proud stood I with my oversize uniform that the Cap'n said I would outgrow before Christmas. 'Any other bugger would fit theirs next Easter' was the last grumble I heard before trekking off to school. In less time than it took to light the first fag of the day one of the negotiators from the third year approached me to announce that a kid called Taff from one of the feeder schools wanted a try out. An image of the Cap'n and my Mother wagging their fingers at me flashed through my mind and I immediately turned the offer down. The playmaker sulked off with the knowledge that his entertainment for the morning had been cancelled. I was stood there thinking of all things academic amidst this mayhem that was going on. Kids were hurling abuse at one another with liberal smatterings of the foulest retorts. My thoughts were all over the place plus I was absorbing the fact that I was walking into an unorganised jungle.

I stepped forward into the boiling cauldron and I was swirled along high ceiling corridors and deposited at the requisite form room. After the introductions of my form tutor I wandered into the main hall and without any surprise to me I was allocated a place in set 1A1. "Top boy", thought I. This was my pre-ordained right but it was probably due to a good school report from the Junior

School. Directions given, orders issued and the first screams of some suited person and off I went. I am Miss Taggart and I am your Form teacher. Normally I would have listened but I drifted off to some place I knew about but had not been to. The ringing in my ears was the bell for break and I was dragged along to the smoker's convention. First up, it was where the hard nuts used to hang out. Second up, if you were the new kid on the block it was your divine duty to have your pockets picked and "crash the ash, young un". I still had a far away thought in my head and I suddenly realised that I was missing the expected first year clip. It had not happened. Nor had my head been thrust down the toilet and flushed. Why? It was years later, when I was in some dingy Rotherham drinker, that out of the gloom an unclassified came up to me and, in an effort to ingratiate himself, he told me that everybody was scared witless of me from the start. Of course, he did not say witless but I took his point.

The morning passed, the growl in my stomach had been appeased for a while and I went off at lunchtime to find somewhere quiet for a smoke. Up he came. Taff and his older brother, accompanied with a few boys who looked like they hired themselves out as professional mourners. This Taff kid was taller than me but slighter build. He had a swagger that would have been comical if it was not for the fact that he approached me mob handed. Once again, the offer was made and the offer refused.

I turned him down and even explained that I did not want my uniform dirty. This was taken by the cardboard gangsters as an excuse that I was frightened. The place and time was set. At 6.30 p.m. in Bradgate Park. Braggie Park, as it was colloquially called, was a park on the opposite side of the road to the school.

At the appointed hour I turned up with two of my mates. No second in command as the summer feud with Big Bob was still on going and the friendship groupings were still divided. My tie had been ripped off to be replaced by a Leeds United scarf and, feeling much better for the wearing of my comfort, I approached the top of the banking overlooking the main park area. Taff was down there wearing a Manchester City hat, looking very confident and surrounded by what seemed to be 150 kids from his estate. Only one thing for it, I thought, and that was to run. Run, yes, straight down the banking and gave him one crack to the chin. Down he went and he managed to twitch his left leg once in half an hour.

The following day, after the Kimmy criers had bellowed their rendering of the story, I became known as One Punch J. Immediate elevation to cock of the year came about without any votes being cast. What a week and it was only the first day.

By this time I had managed to obtain a newspaper round delivering mornings and nights for old Ned who owned the local newsagents. My morning delivery took me through the old Kimberworth village to the site of a listed farmhouse building known as Manor House. My delight was to stroke the neck of a horse called Romany who was stabled there. It was a lovely chestnut with huge eyes. He just loved the sugar cubes that I gave him. However, the evening round was a completely different scenario. My delivery circuit was over the West Hill area of Kimberworth. A third year kid, who fancied himself as a hard mod, took it upon himself to demand one of the evening papers. Imagine my surprise. One week at Kimmy and I was convinced that no kid could read. He obviously did not read my intentions either. A scuffle resulted and I managed to rebuff his demands. The following day, at school, the fight coordinators had put it about that I had been in with a third year notable and upset the status quo. Times and places were discussed and agreed. He thought the time was dinnertime but that is not my way. I run the rules, I make the times. At break time I surprised him and the new found nickname was reinforced. He wore glasses before I hit him but even they could not disguise the blackness that spread over half his face. By the time I arrived to my next lesson after break, I had according to the jungle telegraph demolished him and he was in intensive care. The door opened. It was Charlie, the deputy head and to all who knew better the power behind the throne. "Which one is Tune?" he asked in his affected bored way. I stepped forward like an offering to the firing squad. He wagged his finger twice in a beckoning manner and off he swept with me in tow. At his office he produced a cane and switched it with the expertise born of a county cricketer that he used to be. A double hander was my reward for sorting out an ugly looking kid with specs who had bad breath and crossed my path. Injustice or what? Not to the sadist with the stick. He delivered pain on a scale that I had never encountered. It hurt but the unclassifieds and wannabees in the form were not going to be told that. "Look at that", I said as I proudly showed off the two red wheals on my hands. "Hurt? That? No chance. The guy can't hurt me".

The story soon went round the school that J.Tune can give and take it. My stock rose faster than a hot technology share tip and the rumour control board went into full gear.

As far as I was concerned my number one priority was to do well at school and I made every effort to succeed in my studies. Science became my favourite subject, as it was not something we ever had in the Junior School and it was almost a new world to me. Mathematics was another favourite helped by the fact that the teachers in these subjects were friendly guys who held no power lust. Not like the history teacher Baggy pants but more of him later. Odd thing though, my invitation to join the football team was not forthcoming due to my reluctance to put my head up the sports teacher's crevice like some of the team.

One night I went to the 'Slag Bin' youth club and chatted up an attractive brunette. Naturally, I offered to walk her home for her own safety.

You're my girl, I told her in a very macho way. If the truth be told I was as nervous as anything knowing only too well that a girlfriend was a symbol of acceptance amongst the ones to impress. Did I kiss her? Did I keep my mouth open? How long did I snog her? Whilst I was debating the Casanova moves I was going to make, she grabbed hold of me and delivered a toe curling smacker. Well, that's sorted. A first year boy going out with an experienced second year girl was a result. This lifetime coupling of minds lasted a whole three and a half weeks. Not bad for a number one.

On the back of my turgid love affair and feeling very much Jack the Lad I walked down the drive into school with what can only be described as the Tune swagger. Clenched fists turned outwards, arms by my side swinging slightly and the head going side to side like a hard man's metronome. Straight over to the smoker's corner and there was JoJo holding court. JoJo was the resident number one of the school and when he spoke the rest were hushed. He seemed to be very agitated and he was hopping about from one foot to another. Strangely, his head was going side to side like mine. I looked down and I saw that he was wearing his fighting Doc Martens. "We are going out on strike. These bloody cockroaches do my head in". Cockroaches resided underneath the ground floor of the school, in particularly the two classrooms where JoJo and I had our respective calls for attendance. "So what?" asked an enquiring but slightly brave unclassified. "We are going out on strike until they get rid of them" was the announcement from the leader. The rumour control board took over and within ten minutes the streets of Kimberworth resounded to sounds of protesting students chanting "We are out!" "Cockroaches out!" Most of the staff was trying their best to round us up and herd us back into the school but no one moved. It was ironic really, the cock of the school complaining about cockroaches. We marched off home chanting like a revivalist movement and returned the next day. A deputation came out to greet us and assured us that the caretaker (Vic) had solved the problem. The infamous cockroach strike of '76 is still routinely resurrected amongst the qualifiers of the event. What was this place I had come to? I had made an interesting arrival to Precinct Kimmy. Things can only get better.

After things had quietened down a guy nicknamed Al picked on Steffo. This Al guy was a notable from the second year. He was a singularly ugly looking thing with the usual amount of bad breath to accompany his guttural utterances. I went up to him and politely asked him not to be a bounder and to desist with his activities. When he said "You what?" I replied "F*** off you T*****". Obviously, the refined way of speaking that I had was way beyond him so he offered the both of us out. Braggie Park, at 4.00 p.m., after school. Off we went with what seemed like the whole of the school in tow. 'Fight, Fight' was the cry and it drew a bigger crowd quicker than a girl doing an impromptu striptease. The line was drawn deeper than the line at the Alamo. He was on one side and we were on the other. So, now what, I thought. Who does what? Who starts? Whilst these rhetorical questions were flashing through my mind my fist was connecting with his Neanderthal chin and instantly improved his looks. He hit the floor and Steffo jumped on him and grabbed his lapels. "Don't mess with us or I will finish you for good". What a melodramatic speech from Steffo and, in the strangest of ways, quaint. I let Steffo have the acquired glory but everybody watching knew who the man was or should I say the up and coming?

On my twelfth birthday a girl called Lorraine gave me a birthday card and took me to the Slag Bin Northern Soul dance. All expenses paid by Lorraine including the afters. What a night. My favourite dance music and a girl to take home, what more could I need? We did not go all the way but I kept my hands warm on a cold winter's night in the bus shelter near her house. It did not last long due to the fact that it was soon to be the end of year Christmas dance and there were more fish in the pool. At the dance, there was a competition and I won the event. My soul dancing was improving and so were my pulling powers. Over came a girl by the name of Fully. She was so named because she had a full pair. Well, thought I, the milk bar is open. Merry Christmas and Happy New Year.

On returning to school in the New Year the results of our Christmas tests were announced. I did very well especially in science as I came top of the year. 'A' class again and this was to be the pattern for the rest of my time there. Geography was soon to become one of my favourite subjects to study and it is something that I still obtain great enjoyment from. The teachers were by and large all right. Strict but fair in most things and I still had enough respect for their role in life to keep on the straight and narrow.

At this time my Father was working abroad in Saudi Arabia and, as a consequence, I was spending more and more time with my Mother. Inevitably, I suppose, but at that time I could not see much beyond the immediate, and grown-up ways were not my province then. I helped out with the shopping when I could and kept the garden neat and tidy. The Cap'n was growing older and he was finding it too much of a strain to carry out the things that he used to do. My paper round was the main source of my spending money although my Mother used to slip me the money for the Slag Bin on a Thursday night. She always gave me the same little warning: "Don't do anything that I wouldn't do". Silly woman. As if she would do the things that I intended to do at the Slag Bin. My Mother was beginning to gain a reputation in the neighbourhood for being a woman not to be messed with.

Whilst I was outside minding my own business, my brother and a few of his mates came steaming past me faster than a Kimberworth pupil going on strike. Next thing, this guy known as the Preacher appeared and gave me a right crack on the head. It appeared that my brother and his mates had been hedgehopping and this Preacher guy's hedge was the one in question. Due to the fact that I was a kid and I was there, albeit in complete innocence, I was the recipient of an ex-wrestler's smack. Who was it exactly who told my Mother about this event I do not know but she came round the corner with all her guns blazing. She went up to the Preacher and delivered her brand of a sermon on the end of his nose. He may have seen God but I doubt it as he lasted the whole of two seconds before going down on his knees in prayer of no more wallops. My Mother converted him from the wrathful avenging angel into a whimpering coward pleading for forgiveness. Enough said, we thought, until the boys in blue came round to arrest my Mother for G.B.H. The upshot of it all was that the case was thrown out of court with much laughter from the assembled rent a crowd in the gallery. He was forever dammed and he ascended into heaven or should I say moved from Lower Kimberworth to the top end of the estate?

Chapter 6: The Army Cadets and other Armies

In order to join the army cadets a new entrant had to be one year older than I was at the time. So I backed dated my date of birth to make sure that I was old enough to join. After six weeks of extensive drilling I eventually earned my uniform. We were known as the Kimberworth Hallamshire cadets attached to the Sheffield area command. I attended twice per week and put a lot of effort into it. It helped having some handy boys in the cadets and it certainly was not for the faint hearted. There were plenty of rewards like days out to known attractions such as Flamingo Park, North Yorkshire. The main memories I have of these times were the silly songs that we sang in the back of the Bedford military Lorries. Not so much football chants but songs of love conquests and oversized genitalia.

The main source of money for the boys around town was what was known as the 'weigh in' or mullucking. Either way, it meant collecting non-ferrous scrap and taking it to a scrap merchant for a few readies (pound notes). This was supposed to be scrap metal but it never mattered if it was attached to something. Most of the scrap metal came from old houses in the Masbrough area. Sometimes it came from things that were removed from their original resting places. This was my first introduction to the trade of dismantling. I would take anything apart to obtain the scrap.

Dishonest? Probably. But I was making money and that was all that mattered.

At this time there seemed to be a growth in the creation of gangs. Self-preservation was the name of the game. Skinheads, Punks, Teddy Boys, Rockers and, of course, the Soulies. My affiliations were to the Northern Soul rude boy movement. The difference between a rude boy and a skinhead was that we tended to have a side parting shaved as well as the number one skinhead crop. Naturally, we banded together and naturally we had to have a leader. Nominations were held and, by the process of not being opposed, I was elected leader. The gang was named the Canal Rats. We occupied our own turf, in particularly the Holmes Café. At night, we owned the Slag Bin and any other club that we turned up to. For entertainment, we would turn up to a youth club that was not in our area. We would introduce ourselves before intimidating the boys and entertaining the girls. The dance floor would be ours and so were the girls for the last smooch of the night. Northern Soul music was now engrained in my passions and it has never really left me since.

Our gang was beginning to gain a reputation and the rumour control board at school were soon fanning the flames of over exaggeration. Before long, lower ranking notables would call round to offer their scintillating views on how rubbish we were. It was not long before I thought that some form of remedial action was needed. I say remedial because the guys coming round doing the talking were as thick as the proverbial.

The baiting between rival gangs was gaining pace so it came as no surprise that things came to a head. To my surprise it came in my woodwork lesson. As I was concentrating on the technicalities of wearing the skin off my fingers instead of sanding a piece of wood, a guy from the Masbrough area sidled up to me. This boy used to be the number one boy in his Junior School and only two weeks previously had taken out a Year 3 student in the school playground. When he appeared at the side of me I knew that kick off time was imminent. Sammy, the boy in question, said to me: "You have seen the rest, now see the best". His piercing dark eyes, that were an identifier to his origins, glared straight at me. Again, the question of who is this guy entered my head. Once more, the adrenaline rushed to my head at the same time. No contest. Not with him either. Two seconds after the Lower Kimberworth kiss landed unloving on his sharp beak-like nose, he dropped faster than a dead grouse on the 12th of August. I rubbed my head where it had connected with him and stood back and said a saying I still use today: "Don't mess with the best because the best don't mess with the rest". After the inevitable tickle of the fingers by Charlie, Sammy and I went out to the playground to face the expectant mob. To their surprise we were talking like old friends. Still are to this day.

Not long after this, was the end of year exams. True to form I did pretty well and managed to maintain my place in the 'A' form. The school ground quickly   to a halt for the summer holidays and I am sure that the teachers were glad of the rest, too. They had not encountered the likes of our lot before and along with the strike it was a relief for them to say clear off.

Oh, happy days. That summer was a long one with many sunshiny days. Of course, the Canal Rats were to be found at their favourite haunt, namely the Cut Bank, where the canal meets the river Don. Swimming, running and just lazing about was the order of the day. My friends from the top end of Kimberworth had left my Junior School and had been herded into another local Comprehensive school. I invited them down to have a day with us at the Cut Bank. Unusual, I know, but the defectors had a few tasty girls with them. My party piece was to dive off the top girder of the pipe that went over the canal into the water. No one else was brave enough to do it. Very impressed they were and it was just one of those things that had to be done to keep the J. Tune myth alive.

Alongside all of this I was preparing for the annual army cadets camp held at Queen Elizabeth barracks at Aldershot. To pay for this trip I was still doing my paper-round. As soon as I picked up my papers I read the headlines and then the sport pages. That black day in August I read the headlines that Elvis Presley had died. I rushed to my Mother's house to show them the news. My parents were avid Elvis fans and my Mother was stunned to read the news. The spin off from all of this was that I did not deliver the papers that morning. On my return to the shop old Ned came out of the shop screaming at the top of his voice. One word that I did understand was the word sacked. I showered him with the remnants of the undelivered papers and said, "If I am sacked, you can have the f****** sack yourself". With that I threw the empty sack at him and went. My time was up anyway and my other entrepreneurial talents and outlets were giving me a few readies.

The going to camp day came and I lined up on the platform of the now long gone Masbrough station. My boots were bulled to perfection and the crease in my army trousers was straighter than Sammy was when I laid him out. With great excitement I boarded the train and off we went. Many hours later we arrived in deepest Hampshire and were ordered to attention on the platform of Fleet station. By means of more Lorries than can be seen on a petrol price rise protest we were transported along leafy lanes to our ultimate destination.

We spent a week in camp and all told and each day brought its own adventure. Visits to places like the Ghurkhas regimental home and museum. The day when we went swimming with the regular first Parachute Regiment was an eye opener. These were seriously fit guys but were full of fun and mucked in with us like big brothers. One day we went over the Ghurkhas assault course and this sorted out the men from the boys. On our return to camp we were ordered to put on our full uniforms and to stand to attention outside. For what seemed an eternity, the Commandeer and the Regimental Sergeant Major marched to the front of the parade. The RSM singled me out and marched me across the square to the Commandeer. I saluted him and took one step back and threw another smart salute. To my delight, he announced that I was the best turned out cadet in the inspection. Hours spent polishing my boots paid dividends.

As a treat for my endeavours I was selected to go with the Royal Engineers on a team building exercise. We had to make rafts from odd bits of stuff and cross a lake that was near their camp. It was very informal for the army and it was more like being with older brothers than regular soldiers. It was an everlasting memory and one that fills me with joy every time I think of it.

There is always a down to every up and on my return to camp a kid who had travelled down with us came up to me mouthing off. Whilst he was giving me the jealous fuelled anger routine I was trying to reason to myself why he looked like a toilet pan after a bad bout of diarrhoea. Suddenly, the resentment that had been building up inside of him came to the boil. He had been in the cadets for two years and he had never been singled out for any praise and the sight of me going off for the day was too much for his emotions. He attacked me whilst I was laid on my bed in the billet. Before I knew it he had put three punches into my body and face. Hang on, thought I. This is J. Tune you are messing with. I rolled him over like Tarzan dealing with a crocodile on his day off and came to attention on the top of him. No salutes though, just a quick by the left and that was that. He now looked like someone who was suffering with terminal constipation. His face was red as a beetroot and just as mushy. By 1800 hours he was on a permanent sick parade for the duration of camp.

On the last day, everybody went into Aldershot to purchase souvenirs in memory of their visit to camp. Imagine our surprise on returning to camp to be ordered to open our just packed suitcase. Apparently, the law abiding Rotherham contingent had been on a shoplifting spree. My case revealed no stolen goods due to the fact that I had not pinched anything. The ones who had were dismissed from the cadets. I liked the idea of being in the cadets too much to jeopardise it by silly actions. The fight apart, I took it seriously and I was determined to make a good fist of it. Mind you, I seemed to make a good fist of it with most people. Some more than others.

The remainder of the summer holidays were spent down near the Blackburn Meadows depository. Funny place to be, I know, but this was land of great adventure to us. My newly acquired hobby at this time was rummaging through the waste that was dumped there trying to find the old cod bottles. These were bottles with a glass marble inside that acted as a stopper. What I did not know was that this was the location of an old Victorian dump pit site. I collected these bottles to give to the Cap'n's wife for her to sell at bric-a-brac markets. Of course, she handed me a few bob for my trouble. The black economy was nothing new, especially the colour of me when I had finished digging through the refuse.

The Canal Rats were enjoying the flush of our newly formed status and, as such, we had not really developed a pecking order or rules. Well, they hadn't. I had. But democracy being what it is I had to cater for all walks of life. The lazy days of summer soon drew to a close and, before I knew it, the familiar yell from the Cap'n, "Ah suppose tha wants me t'carry thee to school", was thrown in my direction. So, with some reluctance I dragged on my uniform, poured water over my head as an appeasement to the Cap'n wishes that I was spick and span, rammed a slice of best dripping in my mouth and off I went.

School found me still in the 'A' form but with a different form teacher. His nickname was Marzipan to us ruffians but through mutual dislike I will avoid mentioning his proper name. What caused this dislike you, the reader, may be asking. One day, during the "read a book" lesson, he walked past my chair and gave me an almighty whack on the side of my head. He accused me of talking which was a bit rich as I was sat there engrossed in my book. As it was not the Lower Kimberworth code of honour at the time to grass on anybody, I could only stand up and face him out. I was off, out of the classroom and on my way. Well, going on strike seemed to be the way of it. He obliviously came after me like an enraged bull. Up and down the corridor we went. If music was playing they would have entered us for 'come dancing'. More like the last waltz as both of us ended up hanging on to each other without a handbag being thrown. Big Bob has often quoted the events of the corridor shuffle. According to him, I stood my ground and offered him out. Oh no, I didn't. Even I had enough sense to know that hitting a teacher was just not on. If I wanted to stay in that school I had to pay lip service to oddities like him.

This affair ended up with me being invited to the Headmaster's lair. Of course, he sided with Marzipan and informed me that I was to receive two of the best. With a swishing of the cane like some latter day Zorro, he eventually struck me on one hand and then the other. A bee sting would have had more effect. Somewhat sarcastically, I thanked him for his efforts and went my way. The Tune swagger was in full swing by the time I returned to the next class. I decided not to say too much to the assembled troops who were eager for firsthand information in order to make themselves look important when the smokers' bell rang. I said nothing, merely grinned. Even at this early stage I knew that a smile was a weapon in its own right. Whilst I was grinning I was winning.

In the smokers union behind the annexe block all the rogues of the school used to meet at break times to discuss the days' events. My story had gone before me so the notables of the school offered me a smoke and nodded their heads in a show of acceptance. This was now the place where I went on a regular basis. At this time the number one was Meany Deanie's older brother.

He was not as bad as Meany Deanie and he still stops me for a chat to this day.

Due to moving around Rotherham to different youth clubs I came across one of my Cousins called Tex (Terry). Tex lived in the Spurley Hay School catchment area on the East side of Rotherham. He invited me over to go with him to the school youth club at Spurley. The type of music that they listened to was not my type of music but I put up with it for my Cousin's sake. As is the way of it, I was being sized up by one or two likely lads and it was not long before my Cousin Tex told me that Spurley's equivalent of me wanted to have it on. The negotiators sorted out the place and the time and I duly turned up to the appointed spot. There he was with a crash helmet on. What was that all about? My starter with the Kimmy kiss was out of the question so I converted him from baritone to soprano with one well aimed knee. Game, set and match. As he was laid on the floor I pulled his crash helmet off and told him that there was only one cock in Rotherham and it wasn't him as he did not have one.

The rumour control board back at Kimmy went into overdrive at the news that one of theirs had demolished another school's number one. My reputation was on the increase but there was still a long way to go. The older boys were physically bigger than me but they were only bigger in size, not in heart.

Chapter 7: Birds and Bees

Just before my thirteenth birthday a girl called Sue invited me out. She had already been out with my Cousin Tex unbeknown to me and this was to be a sore point with me as I do not take out family members' women (past or present). As a Northern Soul girl she wore the appropriate skirts for the dances. These skirts had slits in the side and my hands were kept well warm during winter.

We went out with each other on and off for about nine times. In between times she had half the estate and the other half were waiting their turn. The joke was that she walked about with a mattress on her back. Although I bragged off to anybody who cared to listen that I was going all the way, the truth of it was that I was still eligible for church choir service.

She was of course like most women in that she needed wining and dining. A bottle of pop and a bag of chips but it were costing me money. She quickly developed the name of Sue to 'Run-around Sue' just like the song by Dion.

So, I commenced a Saturday job delivering pop with a well-known company. All for the princely sum of four pounds a day. Not bad considering that beer was about nineteen pence per pint at the time.

This extra money came in handy for the Christmas army cadet camp at Proteus, near Clumber Park, Notts. At camp was a guy from Lower Kimberworth called Jez. In the army there is an old saying that if it is not bolted down it goes. When Jez was near anything, bolted down or not, it went. He was accused of pinching out of the lockers in the billets and put on fatigues. Naturally, as I was from Lower Kimberworth, I stuck up for him. Big mistake. I was tarred with the same brush and put on fatigues with him. Instead of eating turkey and the trimmings, we spent our time picking up litter off the floor. Some say that crime does not pay. Not with him, it didn't.

Straight after camp, the Officers undertook a full revue of the situation regarding the Muppet Jez. They instantly dismissed him and I received the hot air treatment from a very loud and course speaking Sergeant Major. Oddly enough, I was told later that they admired my loyalty to Jez but they preferred me to be loyal to them. Who cares wins. I was still in the army cadets and, as for Jez, who cares? He was a loser.

That Christmas marked the last time I ever went Christmas Carol singing. The times change of course. This time I knocked on doors and wished them the season's best. No singing for me. My entertainment skills came with a price. New Year's Eve saw me first footing as the tradition demanded. Face blacked with a lump of Arthur Scargills best and a glass of half finished whiskey in my hand. More loot for the Tuney coffers. One house regularly had relatives down from Scotland and they went mad on the first footing thing. This enterprise was quite a good source of money, especially for me. Good people, the Scots. Never was one for the prejudice thing. An age of innocence was passing and little did I realise it at the time. This really was the time of my advancement and would I turn the clock back to these days and change things? No, I don't think so. I have never regretted anything that I have done. I prefer to let others regret what I have done.

January came and with it gloomy weather and a miserable cold wind that blew straight down the spine and left one shivering furiously. Welcome to 1978 then. Back to school. Back to the drive. And back to the milling mass of the un-teachable by the unable to teach. I soon found myself in my rightful place in the smokers' corner listening to the rumours and half-truths. One of the lads was waxing lyrically about a certain youth club called the 'Chizzy'. It was, according to the mouthpiece, wall to wall with available girls with a set of non-descripts looking after them. So that night I called the Canal Rats to order and told them they could vote to go to the Chizzy. My arm went up and so did the rest. Democracy Lower Kimberworth style. On the Wednesday night, we turned up to the Chizzy mob handed. The mob consisted of two others and me. Run or go in. No contest. In we went. To my surprise they were playing Northern Soul and had tasteful girls. One took my eye and I stared at her for what seemed an eternity. As the youth club had a no smoking policy I went outside to have a smoke. Outside the youth club was this tallish guy by the name of Gilly. He had a flat sort of nose and an unbalanced formed face. He was tall and a bit on the thin side. A bit bony really. "What are tha doin' looking at my bird then?" I replied that I was just looking and nothing more. He obviously thought my comment was a climb down so he called me a dumb c**t. The next day at school, through a cloud of morning break smoke, I related this story and asked if anybody knew him. One of the gofers said that he was a notable from another school. The whole incident prayed on my mind to such an extent that I asked the negotiators to arrange a gathering outside the Chizzy youth club the next Wednesday.

I sauntered up with Big Bob in tow. Well, every commander has his fair share of cannon fodder. To my astonishment, there was a cast of thousands O.K. A crowd of fifty screaming, chanting kids all baying for blood. His or mine, it did not seem to matter. The seconds, thirds and the not counted were discussing where the fight should take place. On the grass bank or in the car park were the main locations up for discussion. I stood there thinking to myself: "Are these idiots for real? It is a fight, not a dance competition". Crack. The first one landed whilst he was stood on the grass bank. The last one landed when he was staggering about on the car park. The Chizzy area has never forgiven me for the taking of their youth club and their number one offering. The myth of Tune was growing and the rumour control board went into full swing.

Back at school my reputation was rising faster than the fodder was falling. Another one gone and suddenly the notables at Kimmy were beginning to look at me in a different light. The original question of 'who is this guy' was changing to a 'when will it be my turn'. Yes, Kimmy was beginning to belong to me and I still had three years left. My elevation to the upper ranks became evident when I realised that I was no longer sharing my cigarettes as people were giving them to me as a hope for securing my favour and protection. Not a bad life this for a second year. My growing sense of glee and self-importance came crashing down one bleak Thursday night when I rolled into the Cap'n's house for my rations.

Chapter 8: End of an era

There was a full on discussion going on in the best room of the house. I was told that I was to change places with my sister Samantha and that I was to return to my parents' house and share a bedroom with my brother Dave. It appeared that my sister was too old to share a bedroom with Dave and this was the only way around the problem. My role as number one cabin boy had come to an end and my adventures on the high seas of the Cap'ns' house were sunk. Back to a crowded house and sharing a bedroom to boot. I know that it was my brother Dave but I had grown used to my own space and it was to be a while before I slept in my own bedroom again. About this time my parents started to have huge disagreements and they eventually parted company. As to exactly why they parted company is something that I have never tried to find out. You explain to me why that's because I cannot offer a single reason for not wanting to know. Too painful? Perhaps. They split and that was that.

I suddenly acquired the unwanted status of man of the house. It brought no special privileges, just being the target for every reason for every failure. Bit like married life then. Mind you, I did receive extra money so that I could go to the Slag Bin every week. Just as well. The Slag Bin was fast becoming my escape bolthole. The Northern Soul music was eating into my soul and I started going to the major venues around Rotherham and Sheffield. Of course, I had to buy the latest fashions to accompany my way of life and this cost money. Money Tuney did not have. Out of the blue the guy driving the pop van who I worked with on Saturdays told me he needed someone for a couple of weeks to help him out. I volunteered my services thinking it was only for two weeks and it would pay for the new jacket and trousers that I wanted. Before I knew it, the two weeks had become four and I seemed to spend more time at work than at school.

My education was beginning to suffer and I found myself slipping down the academic pecking order. I was still in the 'A' form but only just. I could avoid detection, as it was hard for my Mother to keep tabs on me. I started going back to school on quiet van days and I worked really hard to improve my class grades. A balancing act, I know, but what is a 'jack the lad' supposed to do? I couldn't look smooth and be a swot at the same time.

My spare time was taken up with the army cadets and I found that there was not much time to dance, work, study, soldiering and go out with girls. One, from time to time, had to go and the studying caught the cold. Back to the girls and back to love. Did I say previously that an age of innocence was coming to an end? One night, I was child minding for an unmarried Mother of three kids. She came in drunk and said to me that it was time for bed. "No, you pudding", she said, as I was about to turn the doorknob of the front door, "my bed". She might have had a drink or two but I didn't care. Everybody has to start somewhere and I was starting in prime position. She, however, called it the missionary position. She paid me the following morning. Now there's a change to the normal format. "Same again next week love", was her parting words. This, I thought, was certainly a case of looking a gift horse in the mouth, so as to speak. Morning had broken and so had my duck.

This went on for a few weeks but she was who she was. I decided to pass my child minding job onto one of the Canal Rats. Mind you, he had been sniffing around for a while and mates do mates favours from time to time. Keep them sweet. You never know when it is their turn for a return favour.

One night, at the Rotherham Leisure Centre Northern Soul night, I sidled up to a pretty looking girl and awkwardly asked her for a dance. We ended up having the smooch dances and I offered to see her home. I ended up walking her home and missed my last bus. The only thought on my mind was 'what a result'. Her name was Jade and I went out with her for about three months.

This was my first serious girlfriend and I afforded her the status. Every Wednesday night we went to the Assembly Rooms in the town centre for our weekly fix of Northern Soul. We became the Torvill and Dean of the dance floor even to the extent of having made to measure clothing especially for the event. Ours was a perfect relationship and the two of us were regarded as a permanent fixture that would last forever. And so it did. If forever lasts for three months. It ended for the usual reasons. She increasingly went on about my friends and my life style to such an extent that eventually it came down to a straight choice between her or what I was about. Goodbye Jade.

As I shared my bedroom with my brother Dave it was only natural that I confided in him about the break up of my time with Jade. We became very close and I took on the role as brother and protector. In some ways I was determined that he would not adopt my life style or my preferences. The family set up had, by now, sorted it self out. My parents were now divorced but I did not really understand what it meant. I only saw my Mother burst into tears from time to time but, though I held her, I could not really empathise with her. My daily visit to my Grandparent's still brought an undefined joy to me. "Bloody hungry nose is here again", was the usual riposte from the Cap'n. "Yeah", I would reply with a grin on my face. "But what are we having then?" I loved going round there and, oddly, it seemed to be better now I was not living there. Food at the Cap'n's table and back home for some more snap. What a lucky boy.

More and more, my Mother's distress came bubbling to the surface. I was not worldly wise enough to deal with the emotions and hurts, so I increasingly took my brother out of the house with me. One of our favourite things to do was to catch a bus and go to the Sheaf Valley swimming baths in Sheffield for a relaxing swim and more importantly an escape from our immediate environment. Dave, who was a bit of a torment, started winding up an older boy. All I saw was Dave being chased around the swimming baths by this kid. When I caught up with Dave he told me some tale about this youth and about how he was tormenting him. Who knows what the truth was but later, when we were stood on the balcony, this guy came up to us. He was obviously going after Dave and took no notice of me. Wrong call. I decided to introduce myself to him. He needed to sit down and so I dutifully obliged him. He, for some crazy reason, put his chin in the way of my right hand and he was spread eagled in the aisle. My lasting memory of this moment was my eye catching a sign that said 'No Litter'.

That, I guess, was partly the trouble at that time. There seemed to be too much garbage in my life so the cadets became a safe haven for me. My commitment to the detachment grew stronger and I poured myself into the challenges and discipline of the troop. An annual event in the Sheffield area was the yearly competition held at Totley brook. I was a selected member of a team of six representing the Kimberworth Hallamshire army cadet force. My skills as a marksman on the .22 rifle range enabled us to gain maximum marks in that event. We gained high marks in the other events especially map reading, which was my other main strength. It was with bursting pride that we received the military pentathlon cup for that year as we had beaten the other five detachments for the first time in living memory. The only drawback to the weekend was that I had to sleep on the floor of what was known as the chicken hut as there were no spare beds or blankets. Cold was not in it. My pride and joy was the size of a withered walnut the next morning. However, the misery of the night was soon dispelled as I was chosen to receive the cup on the behalf of my detachment.

The euphoria of the weekend lasted for quite a while and I was walking around with the Tuney swagger on parade at every moment. My schooling picked up as well due to this sense of achievement. There was not much to upset my equilibrium and I was firing on all fronts but there was nobody to fire at. My position in the 'A' form was consolidated due to a run of good class tests and I even handed in homework done by me. The wall outside of school was known as the Rank Xerox corner as there was more copying done there than on a photocopier. For a time my secretaries on the wall had no business from me.

The run in to the summer holidays passed peacefully with no mayhem. Eventually, the day that every pupil wishes for dawned and the summer holidays beckoned. For once, I was undecided as to what to do. My Saturday job kept me away from home for one day per week and the thoughts of spending too much time with the Canal Rats did not appeal to me either. So, as I was mad on the khaki, I devoted many hours to improving my army cadet skills. My shooting prowess was improving to such an extent that I was asked to represent our detachment in the 'News of the World' cadet shooting competition.

We reached the final that was to be held at Huddersfield. The final was held over a weekend and our main rivals for the title were a detachment of fifteen/sixteen year olds from Ireland. They were the eventual winners but we gained the minds and hearts of all concerned by being the runners up with an average age of fourteen. Quite an honour and I allowed myself to wallow in the praise that was showered on us. My standing in the detachment had never been stronger and I was quickly promoted to the rank of Lance Corporal.

Quite why I was elevated to the boxing team was never made clear to me. Obviously, someone somewhere thought that I could stand up for a few seconds in a fight. Our first boxing match was held at Strensall Barracks. I was the first reserve and so I thought it would be an experience to sit and watch the others and to absorb some of the atmosphere. Next thing I knew I was in the red corner with a pair of boxing gloves on. The snorting prancing brute in the blue corner was a guy of Jamaican descent who had been in a few bouts. The bell rang and the cadets roared. The fear of losing that I was experiencing made the adrenaline kick in and the shaking in my arms stopped. My boxing knowledge and technique was almost non-existent but I went into the middle of the ring like a raging bull. People told me afterwards that my style was that of a street fighter but to me at the time it was a case of not being hurt and stop the other guy. All he knew was that the traffic lights went to red and he stopped. The referee jumped in and pronounced me the winner. What a cheer. Everyone was on their feet clapping and yelling. I heard nothing and saw nothing. My mind was still in a whirl with the exhilaration of it all and before I could blink I was back in the changing rooms shaking hands with Delroy. He told me that it was a good fight and offered to buy me a drink of pop. This was the start of a good friendship and I have kept a special regard for Delroy. The last I heard of Delroy was that he had a boxing match of his own on Goose Green in the Falklands with the Argies. What became of him after that I do not know and I would love to meet up with him again, but not in a boxing ring.

Two weeks later I was back at Strensall Barracks at York shooting on the .303 range. Through my status as the best marksman in the Sheffield area, I was paired off with a sixteen-year-old called Delaney from Castleford. His Father was an officer in the regular army and he had been brought up in the khaki. He improved my shooting technique and he scored 34 out of a maximum 35. My response was to post a creditable 27 out of 35. His score was far better than any one from the junior leaders could manage and my score equalled the second best from anyone on the day. My friendship with him lasted the all of the time I remained in the cadets and it is to his credit that he ended up as the cadet of all England for that year.

The other notable event of the summer holidays was my mishap when I was swimming in the Greasbrough Dams near Rotherham. Halfway across the second dam I developed chronic cramp in my left leg. That day I was with Meany Deanie and he came to my rescue. I felt really close to him and for a while he enjoyed the shield of my friendship.

As the summer holidays were drawing to a close and the call of the academic machine began I realised that for the most part I had been away from the Hurley burley of Lower Kimberworth. It was with some regret that the process of buying a school uniform for the Third year was now under way as my thoughts and senses were still locked into the cadet way of life. Soon, I was to replace one set of commands by another and one set of mindless screaming instructors by another set. Khaki uniform replaced by bri-nylon shirts and grey Ties with burgundy stripes. Before I knew it I was trudging up the hill to the learning factory. Fag in hand, swagger at the ready. The melody of 'Here we go again' came into my mind. My depression went when I saw that the seething mass stood next to the Rank Xerox wall. Third Year, here I come.

The start of the third year saw the conscripted troops commence their options. One of my options was to join the electronics group. This was presented to the, in Kimmy speak, ones with something between their ears. So, I found myself in the bowels of what was once the R.O.S.L.A. centre. The swots and also ran's were seated around a large square table. This, being early September, meant that the days were still warm and slightly humid. Mr. Mitchell was doing what all good teachers should do and that was to stand at the board and teach the lesson. Unfortunately, the long hours spent on the pop wagon had caught up with me. My eyes slowly came together and I pitched forward in a blissful and welcome sleep. The next thing I knew I received an almighty blow to my right ear. I roared my anger and stood up. All eyes looked towards an excuse of a fighter called Garth. That was enough for me. I launched myself at the intended target and if this had been the Coliseum the scorer would say impersonator 0, the boy 3. Mr. Mitchell did his best to contain me but eventually he ran off for help. The impersonator had a moustache that was so weak that if the wind blew he would be bare faced. I pulled the offending rat hair from his face and kept telling him to shut up, as I did not like the noise that he was making. The place was absolute bedlam by the time the posse arrived with Sheriff Garrett in charge. I was arrested and hauled off for my kangaroo court judgement. Charlie dispensed justice: four strokes of the cane for the hero and two for the loser. As we came out of the make shift courtroom Garth's brother was waiting for us. At that time he was the resident cock of the school, known as Cid. He had heard the story and he made us shake hands and told us to forget it. Until the time of writing I had forgotten the incident. Why be reminded of it? I recently came across Garth at Cid's fortieth birthday bash. That was certainly an occasion. Anybody who has been somebody was there to pay homage to Cid and to drink his pocket dry.

Morning break arrived and I sauntered round to the smokers union. I was singing the words of a Queen song 'Another one bites the dust'. The assembled fag worshippers retorted with 'There is only one J.Tune'. Oh happy days.

School had started off with a bang and I was hoping that the recommencement of the Slag Bin would also lead to a bang. On the third Thursday of the month I donned my finery and entered the hallowed halls of the so named club. O.K., so it was still the same old church hall with decay and yesterdays mould still attached to the walls in place of wallpaper. For the money I did not expect the Ritz Hotel. That was where the female members of the Slag Bin went and we all know what for. I was there for the what for as well. In I went and almost immediately I was pinned up against the pop bar by a bit of fluff. She told me that she had the 'hots' for me and that she wanted to show me her Elvis Presley photographs on her bedroom wall. What the hell the 'hots' meant I did not have a clue but the way she grabbed my pleasure stick gave me some idea. I asked her what her parents would think. She replied that her parents were on holiday and that the house was empty. Off we went on our cultural excursion to view the photographs. I went into her bedroom to have a look at the pictures and to my surprise and initial expectation she appeared at the doorway dressed only in a dressing gown tied at the waist with a snake belt. Whilst she was doing her impression of a vamp I puzzled over her selection of a snake belt. With a flourish that would have gone well in a western saloon she whipped off the dressing gown and said: "Come on big boy". I was immediately assailed by a whiff that reminded me of Grimsby docks on a Monday morning on a hot day. She was waving her legs in the air like an upturned tortoise. I made an excuse that I had a girlfriend and left. I am still not sure I said that or that I did not have a gas mask. Whatever.

This story was not for retelling and this is the first time the story has seen the light of day. I refuse to name the young lady in question, as I do not wish to insult Grimsby docks any further.

Over the next few months I began to wag school more and more. Working on the pop wagon and earning money was of more importance to me and it provided a buffer from the emotions and turmoil at home. I still did not have the strength of life experiences to draw on and I reacted to the problems in my life by choosing alternatives. Call it an excuse or a form of running away from my increasing responsibilities but you cannot put an old head on young shoulders, especially mine at that time. These were not particularly happy times for me and though everyone around me seemed to be wallowing in their miseries no one had any inkling of the anguish that I was experiencing. I could not bring myself to confide in anybody, as the culture of not grassing meant no disclosure on my part.

The reaction to my home life resulted in me taking a somewhat, in retrospect, immature swipe back at authority. My smoking increased and I started drinking underage.

Chapter 9: The never had a kiss gang

Over on the East side of Rotherham were a contingent of relations on my Father's side. Through an invite from one of my Cousins I went to a dance at Clifton Hall in Rotherham. This is where I met members of the infamous gang known as the East Dene Mafia. Flaunting my family Ties I ingratiated myself into their set up. Not too difficult as my reputation had reached the frontiers of East Dene. In my new life I refer to them as 'the never had a kiss gang'. As they were inevitably in and out of jail at the time they never stayed out long enough to have the pleasure of a female's company.

As I was spending more and more time over at the East side of town it was only right that as chairman of the Canal Rats I should call an extra ordinary general meeting and announce my resignation. The teary eyed admirers were further shocked by my revelation that Gasping Gaz was taking over ownership of their futures. In my mind he was the biggest rat of all and it was only fitting that he should be in amongst them.

My time with the East Dene Mafia was a continual round of underage drinking, mindless antisocial entertainment and causing mayhem. One night, nearing Christmas, we heard that a bunch from Sheffield, known as the Pond Street Mob, had invaded the Northern Soul dance held in the Rotherham Leisure centre. This was, as far as we were concerned, a declaration of war. A war council was held and the tactics sorted. In the parlance of the day this was a 'complete liberty'. They were expected back on the next dance night and sure enough they rolled up in their cock sure arrogance, not to mention numbers. We were not daunted by their numbers as we consisted of some of the hardest lads in Rotherham. The trap was laid and they entered it like a hungry mouse goes for the tantalising cheese. They left the centre and we ambushed them like Custer's Last Stand. We went at them from all flanks. By the time the Rotherham police turned up, the street cleaners were out in force collecting body parts and tissue.

Blue lights, wailing sirens and over anxious policemen who were dispensing arrest tickets like confetti at a virgin's wedding was the order of the night. Not wanting to be a paragraph in the local newspaper under the arrested last night column I linked arms with a girl and told her that as far as the boys in blue were concerned I was her boyfriend. "What else?" she asked. "That I have been with you all night", said I. "Oooohh", she whimpered. "I wish you had been". With that, I looked up at the night sky to find my lucky star and took her home via 'the let them have it' corner.

News of the brawl soon reached the ears of the rumour control board up at Kimmy and by the time I sauntered into school the wannabe's were out in full force. Did touching me give them some sense of glory and power?

During this time there seemed to be gangs or should I say groups popping up all over the place with bizarre names to go. The next district on was a place that is difficult to say without spitting so I will leave the name out of it but needless to say there was a cluster of nameless ones wedged together under the banner of the "Braggers". The anointed leader of the 'Braggers', later to be named 'Bradgate mob' was the penultimate cock of Kimmy. This handy lad was who else but Cid. Through a combination of stirring and overloud insults a meeting of the negotiators from the Bradgate lot and the Barkers Park mob took place and the where and when was arranged. The venue for the match was in Barkers Park itself. An away match of some importance. Naturally, in school the next day word went out that all fit soldiers and grunters were required for duty and to assemble at the top of Kimberworth at 6.00 p.m. What an army, thought I. Play the match, win by 7.00 and home for supper. What a shock when we turned up to Barkers Park. There were hundreds of them. O.K. We had fifty and they had approximately one hundred and twenty. Some spotty faced kid with the sort of wart that would make a witch jealous was our membership counter. Up to line stepped their leader called Woko. He was brandishing a penknife in our direction and screaming, "Come on then you b******s". At this point, Cid, who was wearing a long military styled over coat, casually ambled forth and stood looking at Woko. The next thing I knew was Cid opening his coat and bringing out the longest sword that I had ever seen. He whirled it around his head like a whirling dervish. The other lot scattered faster than crows when fired upon by a shotgun. End of match. From that moment on, and even to this day, he was known as El Cid. The only major win of my life without a blow struck in anger. What a shower. They never troubled us again and sunk back into their petty little lives with red faces and wet pants.

Christmas that year passed without incident apart from the fact that I started drinking more and more. My drinkers tended to be the rougher pubs on the East side of Rotherham especially the pub known as the Grapes. This is now a car park for a business but in those days anybody who was somebody had a drink there at some time in the week. The street cleaning machine always came round on a Sunday morning as the streets ran red with the blood from the Saturday night fights that took place. Apart from the fights the other entertainment was the topless girls from Manchester who appeared twice per week and this to me was a joy. Looking at a grown woman's top half was a real treat. Of course, I fell for the all time favourite chorus of "We know where your going", as I went to the gents during a show. That was not so bad but the "And we know what your going for" was faintly embarrassing.

The Grapes was not the sort of place to go in without knowing someone; and I knew the East Dene Mafia. It was a dirty place. Even the rats had stilts on. A huge cave of a place that was always dingy, dismal and dim. This was my venue for a while and I enjoyed the feeling of being one of the lads out for a beer.

I was having one of those weeks where I attended school every day and did not go to the Grapes. My guilt at not going to school took over but by Thursday I was thinking that school was small beer to the life I was leading. Feeling full of angst and impotent anger I walked down my street to see one of my mates. Out of a doorway stepped a fifth year by the name of Scabby. "Uh, Tuney. You are getting too big for your boots. Get on the Stores field and I will sort you out". "What?" thought I, "Middle of the winter and this clown wants a fight" The last thing that I wanted to do was to have a fight but I could not refuse the bout, as he would always be on my back. We reached the field and he turned to me and said, "Come on then, Tuney. Lesson time". Crack. He went down faster than a snowman in summer. "What lesson would that be then, Scabby?" I asked him. He did not reply as he was mumbling to the floor. I left him to contemplate his state of affairs and went home.

A few days later we shook hands, much to the surprise of the rumour control board and the unclassifieds. As far as I was concerned he was part of my immediate society and life is too short to hold grudges. My stock rose another notch and judging by the number of fags I was offered the next day it was obviously a much desired smacking. Even though Scabby and me had shook hands that was not the end of the matter. Whilst I was chilling out at lunchtime with my mates playing football a guy of Italian descent came up to me. He was in the fifth year like

Scabby and he wore clothing to identify himself as a punk. His pedigree was suspect as he was from the Bottom Field Mob at Meadowbank. Without further ado he told me that the Scabby business was not the end of the matter and he head butted me. In Kimmy, you just did not walk away from a scrap, so it was game on. I put my hands up to my head and he delivered two punches in quick succession. At this point I thought I was in for a beating. My old friend adrenaline returned to me and suddenly the power within me welled up. Bang, bang, bang, went my fists as I rained blow after blow in his direction. He wilted under the onslaught and he started to buckle. The challenger was stumped with the next delivery. What a fight. It took me a while to realise that I was not having challenges from kids of my age but from the older and bigger kids who were out for a reputation. Some say that I have been in lots of fights. Perhaps that will be proved to be true but the fact of the matter is that these older boys were effectively bullying me and I was only standing up for myself. Now, in my chosen retirement, I can honestly and proudly say that I have never bullied anybody. My fights have been for self-preservation and not to belittle someone or to take someone out for the sheer hell of it.

The pop business was slowing down and money, or the lack of it, was becoming a problem. To solve my cash flow dilemma I finished with the pop wagon and started work in a Chinese takeaway on a few nights per week. Naturally, when my family came in there were double portions for double less. My Mother was becoming more and more aggressive towards me partly due to the fact she could not order me around like she used to. She resented me being in contact with my Dad and this made her fly off the handle on a regular basis. The verbals were so bad that I felt as if my head was inside a beehive at times. Avoidance was my only tactic during this period but I had to sleep somewhere so I kept my tongue in its place and tried to weather the storm. One casualty was my commitment to the cadets. My enthusiasm had run dry through the continued nagging at home and I decided to put the cadets on hold for a while. Of course, time slips by and my attendance at the cadets ended.

My sanctuary was still the Cap'n's house and he never complained when I strolled in and deposited myself on the settee for the night. Although he complained in his usual manner he secretly enjoyed my visits and still regarded me as a Son rather than as a Grandson. If I could have had my way I would never have left the Cap'n's boat but he was growing older and not up to looking after strays and waifs any more.

In the place of the cadets was inserted snooker. The older boys played snooker with a passion and it was the done thing to follow them into the Y.M.C.A. where the snooker was played. It was a dreary place with torn tables and inadequate lighting but to the boys it was the Crucible and the next opponent was Ray Reardon. The joy of the night was not defeating an opponent but fiddling the timed lights over a table to save 10p and to stop the next players in line from playing. The members of the club were mainly from central Rotherham and the hard core of these were a gang known as the Friday Crew. They played on a Friday thus giving themselves an excuse for an intimidating name to cover the fact that they were just in the top five. Apart from the snooker their main aim was to arrange the where and when for the Saturday home game at Millmoor [Rotherham United Football Club]. The opposing football fans were classified in terms of their potential fighting skills and tactics were agreed accordingly. I could not stand them. Snooker yes but any association with this bunch was strictly not worth queuing off for. After a few weeks of odd stares and mutterings a group of lads belonging to the Friday Crew gathered round me and made it obvious that I was not wanted in the Y.M.C.A. Being me, I shrugged my shoulders and strolled off into the dark. News, however, travels fast and before long the East Dene Mafia got wind of the fact that a gang member had been surrounded by another gang. Enough said. The order went out that gang honour had to be obeyed and satisfied. So, word went out that a meeting of the two gangs was to take place outside Clifton Hall on a mod revival night. The Friday Crew turned up in their finery and were about to enter the dance when my team appeared out of the night. As the Friday Crew had, in a sense, gone up a couple of divisions, this was potentially a tasty fight. My target was a guy called Sparky. He sparked all right, especially when he hit the floor after encountering me.

Promoted and relegated in the space of two weeks. My snooker playing nights at the Y.M.C.A. ended that night and I moved into the main Billiards hall in town. The hall was supposed to be for 18 year olds and above so I immediately felt at home. Before long, the East Dene Mafia took the place over and it became our spiritual home for a few years.

"Jason", screamed my Mother as I walked into my house. "Wagger woman says that you have been skipping school again". To appease my Mother and to stop the melting of my earwax I decided to attend school for the whole of the summer term. Surprisingly, my grades were still holding good and towards the end of the term the teachers were discussing which courses where best suited to me. I found that my name was added to most G.C.E. groups in my options choices. Not a bad result considering the amount of time that I had missed. Makes you think whether schools actually teach anything or just pass the kids' time away. One subject that I opted for was History. The main examination teacher for History was the obnoxious bloke who I have already mentioned. None other than the Minoan like Baggy. Although I did not care for him I did enjoy my map work and the sheer pleasure of reading and looking at the world atlas. A couple of days before the end of term my friend Mick the Bomb was receiving the wrong end of Baggy's tongue due to his appearance. It was not Mick's fault that he was dressed so poorly but at least Mick was clean if not tidy. Baggy kept going on and on at Mick to the point where Mick just exploded in frustrated anger. I leapt to my feet and told Baggy, more or less, that he was out of order. "What has it got to do with you, Tuney?" said Baggy. Whilst he was spluttering that sentence out Mick and I fronted him up. Baggy, being Baggy, chickened out and went off to fetch the Headmaster. We were noted in the naughty book and received a blessing on each hand. I have mentioned this little incident now in order to justify my revengeful act on Baggy in the near future. This was a turning point for me because until this little spat I had regarded teachers with a vague respect that strayed on the right side of pupil expectations. I now realised that they were just people who went to the toilet and did what I did and who had their weaknesses and faults. These thoughts did not stop me from liking some teachers but only if they treated me with some degree of equality and not from an 'I look down on you' standpoint. This awakening realisation has been one of the major strands of my integrity. I have never been a bully and I certainly do not like bullies. Talking down to someone is a form of bullying and I will act accordingly whenever it happens to me or mine.

The school gong went and the collective sigh of relief from everyone in school was heard miles away. The end of term was upon us and off we went. Much to the relief of the teachers and to the joy of the pupils the six weeks holiday had started. Immediately, my thoughts turned to earning money. Within a couple of days I was out mullucking (relocated scrap metal) with a few of the lads. One of the main earners was a guy called Giro Gordon. He had never managed a weeks' work in his life but he knew the benefit system better than the civil servants. He was better at sniffing out scrap metal than a pig in France rooting for truffles. One day, we were after some copper and started sawing away at what we thought was a copper pipe. We were inside a disused house and we thought that we could hack away to our hearts content with no harm to anyone. When there was an almighty bang and a flash I realised that Giro Gordon had sawn through a live cable. He just stood there looking absolutely dumfounded and so was I when the guy from the occupied house next door came in like a bull with a sore d**k. "Well, Olay", thought I. "I am out of here". We ran like the wind and eventually sat down on a small wall trying hard to catch our breaths. It was not the only catch of the day. The boys in blue arrived mob handed and bundled us inside their smelly, body odour filled cars and took us off to the cop shop. As I was technically a juvenile I was dumped on a bench to await the arrival of my Mother. Giro, meanwhile, had been escorted to a cell in the way that only the police can claim happens. Despite the repeated questioning I stuck to the claim that the only reason that we were in the unoccupied house was that Giro had been taken short and he wanted to pass a comment about the state of the world. The police went from me to Giro and back again. Always asking the same questions and always receiving the same answers. The next thing I knew Giro and I were dismissed from the opulence of the cop shop with a few choice comments ringing in our ears. Being a quiet, shy boy, I relied upon Giro to explain to me that 'Off you go you little buggers' meant that the police were not entirely convinced of our proclaimed innocence. By the time we reached Meadowbank we were helpless with laughter. It turned out that Giro had been feeding the police the same story that I was pushing. What a score.

About this time the travelling fair came to town. This was an eagerly awaited occasion and the 'Statis Fair' was always a good crack. The order of affairs was that I would be one of the first to obtain a job on the fair – especially the Waltzer. Well, let's face it; there was money to be made and girls to be made. The girls were known as the Waltzing groupies and they were always up for a free ride. So were we come to think of it. Naturally, they were accommodated. The boys on the Waltzer used to give out the perennial cry of, "The louder you scream the faster we go". I used to shout out, "The louder you scream the harder I go". What great nights they were. As is the way of these things, my prime position as a Waltzer boy came shuddering to a halt. When a customer paid for a ride my job was to put the money in a box that was fastened to the control box in the middle of the Waltzer. Some money went in the box and some money went in my pocket. This went on for a while until a grass whispered in the owner's ear. Jealous guy was the grass. He was fed up with having the crumbs whilst I was having the main course. Well, I am the Tune. The sting was set and I walked straight into it. Hands in the pot so as to speak. I was given the bullet or should I say a fairground way of saying goodbye.

Not that I carry resentment to any great extent but a flair up with some of the younger Gypsies soon happened. As I have said, mullucking was our preserve but the Gypsies started to muscle in on our claim. A few scraps and verbals became the order of the day but day by day there was an increase in the animosity. The anger finalised itself with a full blown fight outside the Holmes Café. Meadowbank versus the travellers. No contest really. There is a lot of talk about how hard the travellers are but they don't meet Meadowbank everyday. The majority of the Meadowbank lads were members of the Canal Rats and I still had a sense of comradeship with them even though my allegiances were with the E.D.M.

In retrospect, this was a nice warm up for the next challenge for my title. I was hanging about with some of my mates from off my estate and we were chatting and kicking stones at each other up by the field gate. The next thing I knew this guy from the Bottom Field Mob called Gammy ambled up to me. He was called Gammy on account of the fact that one hand was bigger than the other. He opened his mouth and snarled at me that he was going to give me a boxing lesson and that I was not like the rest of my family. This joker had thrown tin cans at a few doors and on the strength of this he thought he could be a somebody. Bang! I do hope that he heard me say," If you are going to do it, do it, don't talk about it". I doubt it though. He hit the floor harder than his tin cans hitting a door.

One sad thing about these holidays was the eventual end to the Slag Bin. Not that it closed but I stopped going on a regular basis. As is the way of these things there were younger kids turning up and I preferred to be with the older ones. Why should I have pop and crisps when I could join the lads for a pint and crisps? At odd times I used to go to play table tennis and to tap my feet to the Northern Soul records but only when I was short of cash.

"Tune". "Yes Sir". September again and the start of the fourth year. I always turned up for the first day at least and on this day I found out which of the GCE groups I was in and where they were held. To my delight I was in the top set for English and my teacher was Mr. Price. He was one of the best in the school and I had a lot of respect for him. He worked you hard but he was always fair with his comments and words. I enjoyed the literature side and I discovered a liking for Shakespeare. We were studying Macbeth and I thought it was ironic that here was a great piece of English literature that was about murder, scheming and death. Not quite where I was coming from but no one was going to make a story out of my life. The other subject that I enjoyed was History. We were studying the Second World War and learning about the battles that took place and the causes and effects of the battles. Bit like my life at this time. There were battles every other week with no cause for them but with plenty of effect. History has taught us that wars never really solve any problems but my battles were solving a problem. The problem was that if I did not stand my ground I would be battered. Unlike Hitler, I did not have any ambitions to take over the World. The taking of Rotherham maybe at some time was a possibility. For the time being, however, Kimberworth School was my world and I was determined to meet every challenge to my status as the number one.

One night at the Assembly Rooms dance I chatted up a girl called Jan. She came from the Whiston area and she had the required ingredients: blonde hair, small, with the two hand butt. A two hand butt is where both cheeks of a girl's bum fit in my hands. She was eighteen so I told her that I was sixteen. She was still contemplating whether I was too young for her when I met her outside the cinema. The kid taking the tickets was someone who knew me and he definitely knew that I had not made fifteen yet. Fortunately, he kept his mouth shut but the grin he gave me spoke volumes. Jan decided that I was O.K. so in we went to see a film called 'Quadraphenia'. I have always had a venomous dislike for underage sex but as I was on the receiving end I gratefully accepted the gift. It was no surprise what went on in the back of the stalls in those days. The film was good though, as I found out years later when I watched it on television. She certainly had a sense of rhythm though. She timed just about every move to the music.

We went out with one another for a couple of months until she eventually found out my true age. She forgave me for the lie but her pride was dented. I did not mind as I was eying up another girl at the weekly dance at the Assembly Rooms. After the parting of the ways with Jan I introduced myself to Debbie and I found out that she was closer in age to me than Jan. We were together for quite a while and usually met up three times per week. It was not love but more a status thing. I had a bird, went drinking and played football. What more could I do to enhance my manhood?

I know. Take Gilly's elder brother out. This had been brewing for some weeks and I thought it was about time that we discussed the matter in hand like gentlemen do.

Thursday night and I looked good. Jeans, trainers and the ubiquitous tight Tee shirt complete with the swagger. I was ready, able and more than willing for the evening's business. At seven O'clock the doors of the Slag Bin opened and I prepared myself for the introductions.

When I arrived I found out to my disappointment that he was not there. As I was there I had a couple of games of table tennis and had a long chat to some of the boys. Suddenly, a runner came down the stairs to announce that Gilly senior was on the premises. We met on the stairs and as soon as I saw him I solved both our problems. Mine was the continuance of my status and his was that he could dine out for years on the story of how he went in with me. The open mouthed members of the Slag Bin looked on in awe and the story of the evening events were retold for months after.

For one reason or another my school attendance started to drop off again to such an extent that my Mother was fined twenty-five pounds for failing to ensure my deliverance to Kimmy. With the scream of "And who pays that then, you little...?" resounding in my ears I resolved to do some thing about it. Oh no, not back to school but off to the local window cleaner for a part-time job during the day. Well, a man has to pay his way and that has always been one of my fundamental principles.

When I did pay the school a visit it was like a hero returning home. The unclassifieds flocked around me like seagulls round the incoming trawler. At first it was because I assumed that they were pleased to see me but after a few minutes it became abundantly clear that the chirping flock were being bullied by the last remaining obstacle to my crown. It appeared that the notable of the fifth year was doing the rounds of the fourth years and taking pens, money, even fags off them. The unclassifieds knew that I would not stoop to such lowlife activities as bullying and extortion so they were depending upon me to come to their rescue like the proverbial knight in shining armour. The more I heard of the antics of this Pieman as he was known, the more my blood boiled. Pieman was one of three in the fifth year who were contenders for the number one

112

position. He was taller than me and not exactly a photogenic example. He was, though, quite handy and he had taken out most of the school challengers. At the time, Big Bob had turned up to school following the death of his Father and he was not in a happy state. Pieman demolished Big Bob in the outside school toilets just for the hell of it. When I discovered the truth of this unevenness the switch was thrown in my head and I knew that retribution was going back to the Pieman. At lunch-time I sidled up to the front of the queue and stood behind the Pieman who had pushed his way to pole position. I put my hand on his shoulder and gave him a gentle push. "Get out of the way Pieman, this is my school", I growled at him. He immediately pushed me back but though he had a height advantage on me he felt as weak as a kitten. This cheered me up no end and I knew that I was stronger than him both physically and mentally. A scuffle broke out and a small contingent of teachers ran into the dining hall to break us up. Exactly what was said by either of us I cannot remember and of the time immediately afterwards. My thoughts came into full clarity in the afternoon during my woodwork lesson. The rumour control board informed me that the whole of the school were talking about the forthcoming fight. It was then that I realised that I had not even arranged the thing. "Just going to the toilet sir", said I, as I went from the workshop. I dashed up the stairs to the classroom where the Pieman was sitting. I opened the door and completely ignored the teacher in the room. "Four O'clock, usual place, twat". The door seemed to shut with some force and I could still hear the sound of the door slamming when I was half way down the stairs.

By the time the bell was ringing for end of school all of Kimmy knew that the fight of the century was to take place. How word spread so fast still amazes me to this day.

By the time I arrived at the appointed place there seemed to be more kids waiting than went to Kimmy. The Pieman was there, with a girl on each arm, smiling his inane smile and swaggering like an over confident matador. No preamble; no final words from the umpire; no verbal insults; just action. I strode straight up to him and delivered one of the best punches that I have ever thrown.

People tell me today that they thought it was thunder they heard when I hit him and not the crack of his jaw. The silence of the watching crowd was the thing I remember most. It must have lasted microseconds but to me it was an eternity before the cheers sounded.

The aftermath of this rumble was the elevation of Tuney to number one. As for the Pieman? It was weeks before he came back to school. Apparently his pride took longer to heal than his jaw. A footnote to all this was that the Pieman had been back in school for only two days when Gasping Gaz gave him a good slapping. The Pieman's fall from grace was finally sealed. Although he turned up to school he was a fairly anonymous figure for the rest of his time. The unclassifieds were pleased that the Tune was in charge and a new era befell Kimmy. At least the kids could turn up to school and not be bullied. It did not mean to say that I refused their offerings though.

So what did my status of being number one really mean? For a start I could amble to the front of the dinner queue; I was first in line for the daily gifts from the troops; first pick of all the girls (who was prepared to argue?) and a perceived status within the E.D.M.

Down at the Assembley Rooms I was caught chatting to my ex girlfriend 'Run-around Sue' by my present girl Debbie. Within minutes these two wild cats were tearing lumps out each other literally. There were chunks of hair floating by accompanied with language that a sailor in a bad mood would have been proud of. What else could a boy do than stand arms folded on the sidelines and watch this amazing spectacle take place? Two girls going for it is a frightening sight but at the same time hugely enjoyable. What an ego boost. The end result of this was that Debbie went home and I took up with 'Run-around Sue' again. This was the first time that I had revisited romance and it was certainly the last. It is never the same second time round. Certain ingredients are missing and I cannot help but look at past girlfriends with new eyes. Once they are gone, discrepancies that were previously overlooked now become very apparent. For a romance to work there must be a total acceptance of each other by each other. Faults as well as attributes must be accommodated with the same vigour for it to work.

It was very near to my fifteenth birthday and 'Run-around Sue' said to me that she had the perfect present for me. She told me that her parents were going out for the night and that she would give me my present when I turned up. Bang on the dot I knocked on her door at the agreed time. She opened the door and I was faced with a near naked apparition wearing only suspenders and who knows what. My eyes could not decide whether to stay on her breasts or check out her doormat. The doormat did not say welcome on it but I made sure that I was. She hauled me into her house and attacked me with a gusto that could only be matched by an overcharged nymphomaniac who had been stranded on a desert island for five years. More by luck and not without a small dash of human genetic conditioning I found myself entangled in a swirling mass of hair, smells and groans. To my surprise and manly ego I accepted her welcome with a flourish. Medieval knights could not have jousted as well. The evening ended on a high but low down if you see what I mean. What a score. I felt as if I had truly joined the world of men. At long last I could laugh with the blokes on an even level. I knew exactly what they meant when they churned out their South Yorkshire expressions for all matters sexual.

Needless to say, three days later 'Run-around Sue' was seen on the arm of another bloke. I did not care. My task had been completed to my satisfaction at least. Soon, my eyes were roaming again. I wanted more of this magical thing called sex. The search beams in my head highlighted a likely filly called Terri.

After some time chatting her up with my new found sophistication and guaranteed satisfaction she agreed to meet up with me on the top football pitch of her school. It was dark by the time I led her to the penalty spot for the conclusion of three days persuasion. I scored again. One of the best direct goals I have ever scored. It was only when we passed a street lamp that I realised that there was a white mark on her back. I did not have the heart to tell her but have I laughed since when I think about it.

Christmas was approaching fast and I was asked by interested parties to help out with the proposed Kimmy Christmas disco. Things went well and on the appointed night the disco went off very smoothly. Unbeknown to us, a gang called the Town Mob Gate crashed the disco with the avid intention of taking over. This mob used to hang out in the arcades and other seedy places in the town centre. The heir apparent of this mob was a second runner called Bull. He was a second runner because he was not good enough to join the E.D.M. The rest of the mob, apart from fiddling slot machines and taking money from beggars hats, were a team of has been's and never will be's. This mob ripped the outside toilets apart to make weapons. Once tooled up, they charged the driveway leading to the disco. A now famous goalkeeper was watching the events in his usual languid manner. Without further ado he launched himself at Bull and downed him in one.

No rallying cry here, just normal Kimmy pride kicked in. Bull ended up with a waste bin over his head being pummelled to submission. The rest of the mob soon legged it like the French army at Agincourt. What a set of jokers. It is mind boggling to think that anyone could be so stupid to try and take Kimmy in the late seventies. Even more so when you realise that they were just flotsam floating on the top of the sewers of Rotherham. This was the end of this mob. They disbanded straight after this. How could they justifiable look anybody in the face following such a resounding defeat? Oddly enough, Bull became a D.J. in local pubs. The disco was a turning point for him no doubt. At least he could dance to the sounds of his chosen music and not to our particular beat.

Kimmy school and all who walked her corridors was now the talk of the town. Apart from the E.D.M., who had an age advantage, we achieved a notoriety that was and still is unequalled.

Christmas of that year was the first time that I encountered madness caused by drugs. This was a new and a completely foreign area of knowledge and understanding for me. I had always been brought up surrounded by people who had no time for chemical abuse in any shape or form so I was in some degree of shock and puzzlement. The bush telegraph had kicked in and I was soon alerted to the fact that Gasping Gaz was on one. As I rounded the corner of his street I saw him running up and down the path of his house screaming at the top of his voice. A couple of old dears, who were stood arms folded and clucking like toothless hens, were heard to say, "He keeps going on about the Red W's attacking him". I listened carefully and sure enough he repeatedly shouted, "Go away, Red W's". I would not have laughed if it was not for the fact that he was Kung Fu kicking the imaginary Red W's. It was not long before the ambulance came to take him away. Not before some talkative soul informed me that he was 'popping them' as fast as he could. I nodded wisely without having a clue as to what 'popping them' meant. This was the descent into the Gasping Gaz's hell from which he has never really escaped. Of course, I made the most of it and, albeit from a position of ignorance, I denounced him as a nutter and fruit cake. I just did not know or understood anything about such matters in those days. Prejudice can easily arise through a lack of education and being truly informed. Little did I know at the time but this event was to be played out in a variety of ways during my life. Gasping Gaz disappeared for a while from the Kimberworth area and surfaced several months later on an estate that received its daily dose of lead poisoning from a major highway.

A female friend of mine called Justine asked me if I would baby sit for her one night. I asked her how much for and she said that if I was good boy I would be well repaid. The repayment was just what the doctor ordered and I put myself in line for more of the action. Justine, being Justine, was seeing two blokes at the same time and one afternoon I came across these two having a ferocious argument outside the newsagents. How it happened I cannot remember, but I was dragged into the argument and before long they were both blaming me for Justine's behaviour and attitude. Talk became argument became punches thrown. The first one called Dek hit me in the side of my head. "What the?" I thought. Wallop. Dek hit the deck like a felled tree. The other one, Paul, started to run. Oh no, you don't, thought I. My leap on him resembled a cougar bringing down its prey. A couple of deciding smacks later I stood up. He ran off across the fields like a scalded cat. As I don't paddle in anyone else's muck I baled out. Justine is still friendly with me though and when we meet we always have good crack.

My good times needed funding so I asked one of my Uncles for a job on his ice cream van. A couple of hours on a Saturday soon became all weekend. Of course, I lost no time talking to every available female who came to the van for an ice cream. A free cornet every so often was dispensed with a knowing look and a smile. Who was counting? Not bad for a school kid. Holding down three jobs and studying as well. From an early age I learned that there is no fairy Godmother that will wave her magic wand and make the world better. If you want it, you have to earn it by hard work and application.

By this time, I had dispensed with the Assembly Rooms and on a Monday night and Thursday night I was to be found displaying my stuff in a disco known as Tiffany's in Rotherham. Week by week the place seemed to contain more and more out of town faces. It did not take a genius to work out that the faces were factions of the Pond Street Mob of Sheffield. During the last week of February the place contained more of them than usual. My friend Dydo and I left Tiffany's early, as there were too many of the Pond Street Mob in the place. As we were walking up the road to the town centre a van stopped and the driver, Juddy, one of the E.D.M., asked us how many of the P.S.M. was still in Tiffany's. "Enough", said I. Juddy informed us that a trap was being set for the P.S.M and that we were to take part. Yes please, thought I. Before long the P.S.M. came out of Tiffany's and walked up towards the town centre. A screaming banshee hurtling passed me to take the P.S.M. on. Even in the gloom I recognised him as Speedy Steve, one of the notables of the E.D.M. He managed to take two out before the rest of us charged. From the bottom of the road came another Rotherham group of the E.D.M. led by Pete. The trap was sprung. By the time Rotherham's finest appeared on the scene we had dispersed. The mopping up took hours and it was rumoured that over 15 ambulances were used. That was the last time that we ever saw the P.S.M. in Rotherham although a couple of the guys ended up working the doors on some of the lesser pubs or places where even taking your false teeth out in public was banned.

Whenever it was possible, I still turned up to the Cap'n's house for snap and a chat. Most times it was to listen to their well-rehearsed arguments that were fuelled by three pints of John Smith's fighting water and three bottles of stout. No doubt the extra iron gave her a boost because she always let rip at the Cap'n. The arguments always centred on the Saturday afternoon wrestling that my Grandmother used to love watching. Naturally, the Cap'n, who was very cynical, used to verbally denounce wrestling and anybody who watched it. What a laugh it was listening to these two old crones going at it hammer and tong for hours on end. Even the neighbours turned up to listen to the arguments, as they were so funny. Before long, she would pack her bags and storm off to my Mother's house. Seventy plus years old and she still talked of divorce. How I loved them and how I love the memory of them.

Déjà vu. Another dance and another upset. This time, I was at the Charade Disco with some of the E.D.M. lads. In walked a few black leather jackets who, obviously through stupidity or spending too much time on the open roads, decided to offer us a challenge. When a pint of snake bite was poured over my friend's head it was like a referee blowing his whistle to signal the kick off in a football match. The first blow landed and immediately everybody was fighting. I was tussling with some biker at the top of the stairs when another greaser leapt on my back. Down the rickety stairs we went but not for parlez-vous. Within seconds the whole of the place turned out and the fighting continued on the middle of the traffic island outside the place. As usual,

Rotherham's finest turned up when most of the fighting had finished and threw the injured, knackered or dazed ones in a van and took them to the main police station. Quick thinking as always, I linked arms with a girl and pretended that we were caught up in the fighting. It had worked once for me before and it worked again. It turned out that the bikers were from Doncaster and it appeared that they had not heard of us. They never came back.

School life was still a little spasmodic but I was holding my place in the top sets. I struggled through the end of term mock exams scoring quite well in most subjects. Maths was my top achieving subject closely followed by English and Geography. There is little to tell about this period of school life. It just seemed to pass without incident except for a silly skirmish with one of my mates. Over excitement at the end of a cricket match led to me laying hands on a friend's face. Within minutes we had shook hands and walked home together. This is how it should be. No long-winded grudges or shouting matches. Forgive and forget is not always going soft but a way of letting go and moving on.

The fourth year at school was now over and I was faced with my last school holiday. Once again it was a boy-dominated time full of boyish pursuits with the odd excursion out with some girl. This was a time of innocence that I was never to have again. In some ways these times set the pattern of my life and made me what I am today and the person I have become. The biggest factor was that I became a fighter, and not always through choice, and I have drawn on the ability not to accept defeat and this became one of the main stems of my life. As I am now, I realise that the best form of defence is not to be there in the first place, but naivety and immaturity drove me on.

The summer holidays drew to a close and once again the herds descended upon Kimmy school for a winter's diet of education and mayhem. To the surprise of many, my presence was made known on the first day back and I took my rightful place as the number one. Minor minions called out their greetings to me primarily in the hopes that they would be regarded as cool by mere association. My main objective for that term soon appeared with her mates. I had been tormenting a girl for some weeks during the holidays and here she was in the full splendour of school uniform. Her tie was fastened with the long end first, as was the fashion, so that her knot was huge and the tie barely reached the third button of her blouse. My eyes could not help but look at the end of her tie whilst my imagination and lust went in different directions. This was a seriously good looking girl who, if the law of the jungle was applied, should be on the right arm of yours truly. Her mates were nudging her and pointing in my direction. It was obvious to everybody that an undefined chemistry was going on and it had nothing to do with Science lessons. For the next few weeks I wasted no opportunity to be wherever she was even to the extent that I played table tennis near to where she had her gym lessons.

My interest in her extended to walking the long way round to my house so that I would coincide with her route home. For a change, she was a small, good looking blonde haired filly with a brain and humour that exceeded the usual Kimmy offerings. My conversations with her seemed to be very stunted and afterwards, when I reflected on what I had said, I always regretted not saying other things. The main reason was that she knew my past better than most and all I ever talked about was my previous escapades. For once, my normal bravado and cockiness was at complete odds with how I was feeling. Puppy love? Most definitely. Trouble was, I was not prepared for it and in my immaturity I bungled my way from one stance to another. Never quite saying the right thing; never quite acting in the most desirable manner. Being number one of the school had its responsibilities and mooning around like a love sick Romeo did not rest easy. Whilst my egoism was forcing itself to the fore I was slowly losing a girl that I had fallen for. Of course, I was in love but I just did not know how to handle my emotions. What was I to do in such circumstances? The answer came in the form of some toe rag called Deano. He was an up and coming martial arts devotee and he had been moving through the ranks at some pace. At this time, someone had wrecked the school toilets, so in order to use them during class time a pupil had to have permission to borrow the key from the office. Bit embarrassing if someone was in there for longer than a cigarette. Naturally, the school as a whole was annoyed and so was I for not knowing who had done it. Vic, the school caretaker, pulled me to one side and said that he had heard from a good source that Deano was responsible for the toilet damage. I have always tried to have at least two sources of information feeding me the same story before I acted upon so I bided my time until I had made sure. The waiting time was suddenly reduced when Deano started to brag about what he had done. His comment of "What's Tuney going to do about it?" was sufficient for me to go looking for him. I caught sight of the blustering clown outside the school gym at the start of lunchtime. He took his jacket off and motioned me over to him. The crowd parted in deference to the king. I walked up to Deano and with hardly any back swing delivered the Tune form of justice. He crumpled to a heap on his jacket and I thought that at least it stopped him becoming dirty.

Later, I tried to explain to my heart's desire why I had been involved with Deano. J-J was not at all sympathetic to my cause and I felt that I was losing her without ever really having her. She explained to me that although she liked me a lot she could not handle the notoriety that went with the territory. This threw me somewhat so I decided to calm down a bit and concentrate on my schoolwork. My attendance was impeccable and I made serious inroads with my examination projects. I had to do something to win J-J over and I had rationalised that this was the only way.

Needless to say, what I did outside of school rarely went back to her.

One night, after a night out at Tiffany's, I caught the last bus home to my place. There I was, sitting on the back seat like ten men, when a guy known as Eggy came up to me and told me to move. "Are you talking to me or chewing a brick?" was my immediate reply. One or two people sat near me tried to hush me up and they told me that it did not matter. Not to them maybe, but this is J.Tune. He lunged at me with his fists flaying like a thresher in the cornfield. At that moment the bus went round a corner and he was thrown to one side. Kick off time, thought me, and so it was. I grabbed hold of him and tossed him up and down the aisle like a bridegroom who cannot make his mind up. This Eggy guy was twenty-one at the time and he had a bit of a reputation as a football hooligan. Much later, he was given a five year jail sentence for super-gluing an old ladies hand to a freezer whilst he ransacked her bungalow. No regrets. When J-J heard the story from the bush telegraph service she agreed with me that he deserved a ragging because of his age and because it was self defence on my part.

Back at school, one of my favourite lessons was a road safety lesson that included learning to ride a moped. The lessons were held on the playground away from the main school building. As soon as it was my turn, the Tune exhibitionist side came to the fore and I started to show off. Of course, I fell off in an untidy heap much to everyone's amusement. As I slowly pulled myself up the laughter diminished and the lads began to find more interesting things to look at. The only person who spoke was my friend Doug. He asked me if I was all right and I duly nodded. It was only later when I recalled the incident that I realised that even Doug was laughing his head off at me. For once, I just smiled to myself. Doug has been one of my most trusted friends over the years and I regard him as a brother. The crack that we have when we meet is worth the entrance fee for anybody who listens in on our conversations. He can tell a good story when he has a mind to but he never embellishes a story in order to make it sound better.

Another good friend of mine from Lower Kimberworth is a guy who has always been known as Tez. His Mother used to make the most delicious dripping sandwiches with lashings of Yorkshire relish and enough salt to preserve a cow for winter. Tez and I were returning home from an evening's excursion and we were walking through our estate when a car containing four men pulled up along side us. The passenger window slid down and a gruff voice asked us what we were looking at. "A pile of mobile shit?" I replied. The doors opened and out piled exactly what I thought. Tez and I stood back to back like heroes in a war film and the action took off. My old friend adrenaline visited me once more and I let rip. Fists flying, punches thrown. Exactly what does happen in a fight is anybody's guess. All I know is that self-preservation coupled with a desire to stop the other guy is what motivates the action. Three down in seconds and the fourth guy took off as an Olympic medal was waiting for him round the next corner. Tez and I hugged each other and burst out laughing. Only recently, Tez recited this story to his Son in my company. I just smiled and vaguely nodded my head. It is different in this present era. This is not an age in which to impress anybody. I prefer to use my brains not brawn.

But, and there is always a 'but', those days were not now and I still had not reached my sixteenth birthday. When the great day arrived I decided to go baby-sitting with J-J but she did not know that it was my birthday. After the kids were tucked up in bed we sat on a settee listening to Elvis Presley records. I decided to tell her that it was my birthday and she grabbed hold of me and started to kiss me. My total respect for J-J prevents me from saying more about that night and if you, the reader, feel cheated so be it. My relationship with J-J went up a gear and I thought that nothing could destroy the happiness that I now had. What I did not bank on was life always has a habit of handing out reality checks and my next jolt was soon in arriving.

The other major Comprehensive School in the area was making noises and their resident number one had thrown the gauntlet down by ripping up the schoolbooks of one of my female friends who went to the same school. She said that she was a friend of mine and he more or less dismissed me with some withering barbed comment. Not soon after this slight against me I rounded up some of Kimmy's notables and caught the school bus that went to Kimberworth Park. The school bus went near to the other Comprehensive School. Pip, an upper school pupil of the said Comprehensive, gave our school bus the two fingered greeting. Someone on the bus rang the bell and the bus quickly ground to a halt. We piled off and walked towards the school gates. I adopted the J.Tune stance and shouted out, "Come on then". Their resident number one came out to meet me with an affected bravado. As soon as he was within strike distance I greeted him with one punch. He fell to the ground and remained motionless. I moved off to the nearby cemetery and observed the comings and goings.

An ambulance appeared along with the boys in blue. After what seemed an eternity, he moved a leg and eventually made it to the ambulance. What a relief. I was somewhat worried that I may have caused him serious damage. The next day I was on the school playing field in my football lesson when one of the P.E. teachers told me that I was required in the Headmaster's office. When I arrived the room was full of people in particular the Father of the defeated one. He had a hate tattoo on one hand and a love tattoo on the other. He began to mouth off at me and he told me that he was going to sort me out with his Son. Without further ado I gave him the Kimmy kiss before anybody could stop me. As soon as my head butt was delivered I said, "If you are going to do it, do it, don't talk about it". With that, I strode out of the office. I spent the next few hours waiting for the inevitable call to Charlie's office for the cane. It came to my attention that because the love/hate guy had come onto school property without so much as a by your leave it was his fault that he ended up on the deck. The teachers were secretly pleased that I had pulled that one off and they made sure that no further action was taken. My hero status in school reached new heights and I was now the undisputed number one of the whole area. This story still does the rounds when the boys of my year meet up.

Chapter 10: School's out forever

Just a little more preening was needed with a small splash of something out of a green bottle. Not too much, as my reputation as a rude boy was not to be endangered. It was almost time to go to the school Christmas dance and the prospects of dancing with J-J filled my inner soul with pleasure and some desire. The brogues were given one last wipe on the back of each trouser leg and I was ready. By the time I made my entrance the school hall was a mass of gawky bodies trying hard to look cool and dance even cooler. J-J came over to me wearing a face like solid granite and a mood to match. Every question that I asked was met with a monosyllabic retort. Eventually, my good mood changed to one of questioning anger. Eventually J-J blurted out in response to my enquiry "Have you got the face on or what?" that she was seeing someone in the Marines and that she fancied him. I was devastated by this knock back. Considering that I was willing to fight grown men the hurt that hit me was unbearable. I just did not know what to say or do. The macho part of me prevented me from pleading with her but my heart was screaming out in pain and bewilderment. I spun on my heels and stormed out of the hall eager to remove myself from the whispering throng that looked liked extras in a soap opera. I apologise to the owner of the dog that I kicked and to the owner of the dustbin that somehow fell over. My lungs eagerly sucked in the nicotine filled smoke and I exhaled loudly and coughed. If anyone heard me, it would be my excuse as the truth was that I was close to tears for the first time since when? The remaining days, until the start of the festive season, seemed to drag by in a slow moving meaningless manner. When the bell rang to signal the release of the Kimmy swarm for their annual excess little did I realise the bell was the last school bell that I would ever hear.

What did I learn from the trauma of the J-J break-up? Should I have talked to someone instead of bottling it up inside of me? Should I have stayed at the school dance and pull another girl? What tactics should I have used?

In my new life I look back at the events of that Christmas dance and ask myself what the hell was that all about? At the time I did not have the experience or mental tools to hand to deal with the rejection. I buried the feelings inside a safe that was hidden in the furthest corner of my mind. Although I thought that I was handling the affair, the toll of the loss of J-J, trying to catch up with my schoolwork, the disparity of my home life, working long hours and a lack of sleep was building up like a subterranean fissure. I was like a tinderbox ready to go off and it required the smallest of sparks to ignite the igneous vapour in my head.

During the holidays, I went off with some older lads for a few beers in a local drinker. I was holding my own with the beer and feeling quite in control of myself. The beer took its normal natural course and I shot off to the toilets to pass an offering for Blackburn Meadows. When I returned to my table the lads were in a giddy mood and I could not tune in to what the joke was. Odd comments would be made immediately followed by raucous laughter with me feeling like a complete outsider not understanding the in house humour. Down went the remainder of my pint and I sat back in my chair as a sudden rush of light, buzzing and disorientation hit my head. All feeling went from my limbs and the voices of people seemed to be miles away. Faces swam into view and disappeared again. "Another drink then J?" asked one of my mates. I shook my head slowly but the swirling continued. I had not felt like this since I was five years old and sitting on a fast moving roundabout in the local recreation park.

Memories are fine when the brain is clear and events happen in their logical order. On that night events were random and my reactions were random too. One minute I was sitting peacefully at a table, the next I was belting the life out of some bloke in the pub car park. I meandered my way back to the pub and a flash of pure blinding light hit me nana-seconds before a thudding pain. The hurt was the result of some fella hitting me with a stool just above my right eye. I staggered and weaved my way down the car park to the main road. During the night I would have flash backs of the evening in the pub but every time the running order would be different. The following morning I walked back to the pub to have a word with the land-lord. The bleeding from my head wound had slowed to a thick dribble and I kept a cloth pressed to my cut to mop the oozing blood up.

When I arrived at the pub I started to ask the land-lord a few questions. I was rational, quiet and above all polite. When the boys in blue turned up the land-lord accused me of shouting and swearing and issuing threats to everyone. This galvanised me into action and I resisted any attempts to arrest me. Not for long. The next time my mind stopped and peered out at the world through my bloodshot eyes I was in a cell with a policeman removing handcuffs from my wrists. A doctor was summoned and he told the boys in blue that I needed medical treatment for my head wound. Somehow, I had given them my name, address and age and, being a juvenile, it was a priority for me to receive treatment. The handcuffs went back on again and my mind told me no to that one. By the time my mind stopped again like a wheel of fortune, with a definite click and on the losing number, I was sitting on a hospital bed having stitches in my head wound. On my return to the house of the unwashed my Mother was waiting for me and she told me that I was to be charged for various offences including assault, resisting arrest and causing an affray. I did not understand. Desperately I searched the depths of my mind to remember what had happened and for the love of God I could not visualise anything apart from the pub car park fight.

My Mother took me home and that night was spent with me in a complete daze listening to music and, so I have been told since, rambling incoherently for hours on end. Early in the morning, an ambulance turned up to the family home and I was ushered inside. I thought that I was going back to hospital for my head injury but in reality the purpose of the ambulance was to take me to the psychiatric wing of the hospital. The ambulance turned into the designated bay and I saw a sign pronouncing what part of the hospital we were at. What a stigma to be brought here. On top of that, I was frightened to death. As soon as the doors of the ambulance were opened I took off like the hare at a greyhound race. Just like the hare, I was caught and hauled off to the most depressing room I have ever seen: a mattress in one corner smelling like the unclean corner of a football stadium's gents' toilet, a cardboard bed-pan, and a cardboard urine bottle in the other.

I stared at the door and wondered if I would see the outside ever again.

So, what happened that night in the pub? My Mother always maintained that someone spiked my drink when I went to the toilet. The results of the hospital stated that there were traces of an illegal chemical in my body. I know for sure that I never had anything other than beer that night. Whatever it was it certainly accelerated the turmoil that my mind was in.

The name of the person who spiked my drink has never become public knowledge. One of the people in the pub that night was an old adversary of mine and the finger of suspicion has remained pointed in his direction since that night.

I admit that I was close to a breakdown but the introduction of some unknown chemical tipped the fragile balance between knowing and mental escape.

My perception of the reasons for having a breakdown is that the mind goes into protective mode and shuts down long term and short-term memory functions in order to protect the mind. The absence from reality prevents visual or thought induced triggers that the mind finds too difficult to cope with. Stress is often generated by the mind trying to juggle too many demands and consequently fails to allow the mind to address the more pressing issues. Throw in an emotional firecracker and the move from stress to breakdown could happen in an instance.

Chapter 11: Legalised Submission

Whilst revellers were bawling out their insincere wishes I was heralding the start of 1981 in a Spartan room dressed in stiff pyjamas and sporting the most fetching of foam slippers. The question 'what' came to me as a prefix to every doubt or thought that I had. What was I doing there? What was it all about? Day after day an apparition in white offered me a cocktail of drugs and tablets. They called it medication but to someone who had been brought up mainly by old people I still clung to home made remedies and I was not ready to put my trust in a pink pill and a beaker of brown coloured liquid cosh. Eventually, my refusal to take the daily tranquiliser resulted in me being thrown on my stomach by the largactil squad, who consisted of the largest personnel they could find and being injected in the left hand cheek like an egg fertiliser kit. The only difference was that I never became pregnant only impotent for a while.

My days on the ward were spent walking wearing nothing but pyjamas and foam slippers; drinking water like there was no tomorrow. No one bothered to explain to me what was happening or why I was there. Perhaps they thought that I would not understand and possibly kick off. I perceived that I was on the Psycho Ward and I did not belong there. Long after the results of the spiked drink had disappeared I was still wandering around this ward like a ghost trapped in a haunted house. Days came and went with little to break up the monotonous routine of the nurses. Like a Pavlov dog I would dribble when it came to medicine time knowing that food would come along shortly afterwards. It was only when a shaft of bright sunlight hit my eyes that I realised that I had been in this place for over six months. My school mates had taken their certificates of failure and were preparing for their great life adventure when Kimmy school tipped them out for a life time of dole or some other meaningless pursuit.

My discharge came soon after the school leaving day and I duly collected my meagre belongings and said my farewell to the residents. I said goodbye knowing that all they were thinking about was when is it food time. My Mother came for me and I went into a dream like state whilst she talked non stop all the way home. At least I could wear proper pyjamas that did not stand up on their own in a corner.

I cannot say how much I appreciated being back home with familiar sounds and smells. How often do you listen to a washing machine and Elvis Presley at full belt and not hear any of it. They are everyday sounds that mean home sweet home. My days were spent mostly in bed spooning feeding myself with a cocktail of medicines that some white coated genius in an unknown lab had put together. Would the expert know that the recipient of his/hers daily work was helping me through my traumas. Unfortunately for me I began to depend on my Mother to give me the correct dosage at the right time. She decided that this would be a good time for her to undergo a difficult period and it was certainly a case of the 'out of it' leading 'the going into it'. Between us we managed to turn the corner and after a few months I felt a difference in my well being. I was well enough to eject myself from my bed and try a few steps around the house. This was usually done when my Mother went shopping and so it was that I tumbled out of bed for a gallop along the landing and a skip down the stairs. Unbeknown to me she had forgotten her money and she returned to the house just as I was tentatively making my way down stairs. "You conning little ****", came a full pitched cry. For any one coming out of something that resembled Cold Turkey they would appreciate the complete lack of sense and mental disorientation that I suffered at that moment. A combination of weeks of a haphazard medicinal intake and a lack of misunderstanding on my Mother's behalf eventually resulted in her going to the doctors and having a surgical confessional about the world's ills. The doctor came round to the family home and gave me the once over. He suggested that I should consider being readmitted to hospital so that I could be given a full course of treatment and bed rest. It was more to do with a having a relapse through incorrect applied medicine than a recurrence of my original reasons for hospitalisation.

A nurse, of German descent, assisted me with a bath and spoke to me in a calm yet professional manner. She was a change from the menagerie of hospital staff whose preference was to use drugs as a means of making their job easier. Her kindness in the midst of indifference was something that I will never forget. In many ways, she was a for-runner of the modern techniques in use today.

In November, six weeks into my second stay at the Rotherham Royale, I encountered a Dr. Parker. He was a Consultant Psychiatrist who resided in an office rather like a Headmaster in a Comprehensive School. In a scene reminiscent of my Kimmy days I sat at the pauper's end of a huge desk answering the rapid questions that were being fired at me. In order to entertain myself I decided to ramble on about the qualities of magic mushrooms and what benefits they could bring to my life. He asked if the mushrooms were an integral aspect of my daily routine. There I was, aged sixteen, being asked a question that someone with further education would have difficulty discussing, being expected to give a thesis in response. I was, of course, talking a complete load of nonsense but this guy brought up on a diet of cause and effect peered at me through his half moon glasses, scribbled his undecipherable hieroglyphics on a prescription pad and waved me away with a limp wrist action completed with a disinterested snort.

The result of this interview was that I was now prescribed drugs to counter act my perceived hallucinations. No matter what I have done, I have never hallucinated in my life. It was clearly my fault that Dr. Parker arrived at his conclusions but at that one moment in time I thought it was immensely funny. I decided, instinctively, to go along with this misconception that I hallucinated and smiled my smile behind the backs of all concerned. Little was I to know what the repercussions would be of this seemingly unimportant episode.

I trotted back to the ward resumed my place in the bed that for some reason had my name emblazoned across the top of it in big letters. I threw myself onto my bed and laid there in the classical pose with my hands behind my head, whistling a non-descript tune to the ceiling and with my feet crossed. After a while I reared up and took a good look around the ward. There were a few new comers in the Dormitory (Ward) including a tall, slightly hunchbacked, spindly sort of weed peering at every one with bird like eyes through glass bottomed glasses. He kept on muttering religious quotes and retelling the virtues of God and Jesus Christ. Eventually, he crabbed his way over to my bed space and shuffled on the spot like a tired line dancer. He obviously had something on his mind so I asked him to spit it out or remove himself. He half smiled and began to tell me what he used to like doing. At the point where he told me that he would stand outside the school railings eyeing up Junior School children my acknowledgement that he was no more than a raving nonce rang in my head. Of all the crimes against humanity the worst is crimes against children. Any suggestion of violating a child

142

makes my blood run cold and feelings of repulsion sweep over me like the ebbing tide.

As this creature was warming to the subject of touching little innocents I stood up and hit him with all my strength. He shot back and banged into the bed opposite me. The alarm sounded and the largactil squad poured into the Dorm like the S.A.S. on a mission. Despite my protestations I was dragged down to the seclusion room and once again the peashooter was used to fill my body with legalised submission.

I thoroughly denounce nonces and they have no right to be in society at large. I had no regrets as far as my reaction to this insufferable wretch but on reflection I should have reported him. Whilst I have always maintained my stance of never grassing I will advocate that where paedophiles are concerned it is more than acceptable to report their activities or intentions to the authorities. It may be that the hospital staff where not aware of his leanings and I should have used alternative tactics to raise awareness. On my return to the ward a few days later I noticed that the said nonce was no where to be seen. The ward 'see all' told me that he had been removed, horizontally, from the ward and sectioned in the bowels of the hospital. As far as I was concerned it was not the bowel he should be going in.

Back on my bed, whistling my non tune, I thought that peace had descended upon me and that lightening could not strike twice. No accounting for the weather condition called reality. I had taken to chatting to a guy who stood six feet four inches tall who used to tell me that he was an educated man and that he could help me with my maths. So it was that just after the supper drinks had been served that I drifted over to his bed space. He was in bed with the sheets tucked under his plump double chin. His head nodded in the recognised manner of fellow conspirators and I went closer. With a leer on his face he whipped back the sheets and pointed to his now erect penis. In a hoarse whisper he told me that it was not puffy if I finished him off. I finished him sure enough. I lifted him and the mattress upright and he landed on the floor face down. He was still there when the largactil squad poured into the Dorm again and hauled me off. He remained on the floor like a discarded drawing pin that has been trodden into the carpet. Once again, on my return to the Dorm another one had disappeared. That was the one and only time that I have ever been propositioned by a homosexual and hopefully the last. I do have a live and let live attitude but my manhood goes in one direction only as all the girls will tell you.

Life was not all bad on the Psychiatric Ward. For a starter, the fodder was exceptional and to someone like me whose stomach was always growling this was food heaven. It was normal for me to go round the food servery in the dining hall twice in one session. No wonder my frame became larger. The discos held every Wednesday night were the highlight of the week. This was an excuse to spend hours looking my best and quite often my sister Samantha would come up for the evening and stay with me listening to the latest sounds from the hit parade. I also spent time in the small keep fit gym attached to the unit. Before long I was using the top weights with little effort. During the three months that I was in there my body shape altered due to a combination of good food and regular exercise. Bit by bit I settled down to the regime and I slowly learnt how to play the game. By the time I had turned the corner, and the possibility of my discharge was being discussed, the impending court case for the alleged assault against three police officers now arrived.

I went to court with my Mother and met my solicitor for the first time. He briefly looked at his notes and advised me to plead guilty. My Mother told me to keep it simple and not to volunteer information. The court had received a report from Dr. Parker and the Magistrate based his decision upon the information from the hospital. The upshot of it all was that I was given a two year supervision order under the Psychiatrist and the Probation Service. This was certainly better than a possible four year stretch in borstal. My discharge from the Psychiatric Ward came into effect and I was requested to attend the outpatients every month. Thus, on the fourteenth of January, 1982 I strode out of Rotherham hospital and straight into a probation house in the Eastwood area of Rotherham.

Chapter 12: Probation House

The probation house contained three bedrooms and I was assigned the box room. The other two bedrooms belonged to two brothers by the name of Trevor and Bill Peacock. These guys were ex-borstal/jail boys and big cannabis smokers. Before long, through consistent questioning and a little detective work, they found out that I had been in the Psychiatric Unit at Rotherham Hospital. As it was still a huge stigma at the time there were always references to the 'nut house' or jokes about 'nutters'. Weekends were the worse for this as they would invite their mates round for a smoke session and a few beers. Before long, the crowd would start their funny farm jokes and I became increasingly isolated. I spent more and more of time in my box room to escape the tormentors. My school friends never paid a visit and I probably did not want to see them during this time. Apart from a weekly visit to the Cap'n's house for Sunday lunch I spent my time in my box room as a recluse. I was just not right at all. A lot of will power had left me and I felt bereft of the skills to combat my moribund state of mind. In short, the system had deserted me. No after care or counselling just fend for your self and get on with it. Help!

Amongst the many floaters who turned up to the house for their weekend fixes or just for a place to flop was a friend of the brothers called Jud. As the weeks went by I started talking to Jud about my situation and to my surprise and joy he was very sympathetic. We used to play cards or monopoly to pass a few hours on and I began to look forward to seeing him. After a while he invited me to spend an evening with some of his mates and family and bit by bit I increased my circle of friends. My own family had given up contact with me during this period and so did most of my so called friends from Kimmy. I really was not looking after myself to such an extent that depression set in once again. Weeks of eating junk food, feelings of insecurity, low self esteem mixed with an over whelming sense of detachment from the normal routine of reality took its toll. The final release of my pent up anguish came on the night that the two brothers, in a drink fuelled rage, decided to have a knife fight. No wonder I viewed the proceedings with such a feeling of complete misery.

I locked the room of my door and made my way back to the hospital. The hospital admitted me without the slightest hesitation and I spent Christmas of 1982 sitting on the same bed as before surrounded by the same people. Despite the depths of despair I was suffering I also realised that as far as the other patients were concerned I had never left the ward. "Is it Christmas", said one patient. "Yes", said I. "What year"? Roll on!

One of the guys in the ward was known as Zippy. He was called that due to his frequent tendency to slash his own throat. This man was a total weirdo even by the standards set by the other patients. Late in January, '83, he approached my bed and in an even voice calmly told me that he would open me up like a 'Sardinia'. Poor bleeder, he couldn't even say the word right. I thought long and hard about this invitation to become a second Zippy and after two seconds dropped him with one crack. Within seconds I had legged it out of hospital, not wanting the largactil injection squad paying me a visit. Not one for overdosing during the day, good boy that I am. On entering my house I was immediately hugged by my brother Dave. He peered over my shoulder and I heard him say something about being good to him. I spun round and to my surprise a policeman was standing next to his panda car. Obviously, the hospital had informed the police of my unscheduled home visit and had arranged for a black and white taxi to take me back. The policeman quietly said to me, "There are two ways of doing this. Either the hard way or a way to suit me". He instructed me to finish the cigarette that I had lit up and he waited patiently whilst I finished a cup of tea that Dave had made. He opened one of the back doors of the car and asked me to get in. No handcuffs, just a quiet talking bloke who treated me with some respect and courtesy. The heavy handed approach does not, and I doubt if it will ever do so, work with depressed or dysfunctional people. If you were rushed by a number of people shouting at you and trying to handcuff you, would you give in meekly and say thank you afterwards?

Chapter 13: Back Again

Although my medication was increased slightly I did not become the target pin cushion for the largactil squad. No gold medals at the Olympics for this event. Back on my bed I surveyed my kingdom and relaxed to the banter of the never ending and often repeated conversations that took place. As for Zippy? He became my table tennis partner in the Occupational Therapy Unit and we remained unbeaten to the day I left.

  As my medication began to do its job my mood changed. Confidence slowly flowed back through my veins and my general well being started to improve. One of the side effects of my progress was the realisation that sex had been put on the back burner. It would not be long before that aspect of my rehabilitation was put right. In the Day room there was a girl called Gaynor sitting opposite me. With a lopsided grin on her face she parted her legs and treated me to view that only a Gynaecologist should look at. Following the command of a nod of my head she followed me out of the Day room and into a small dark room down a side corridor. With my jeans around my ankles like a small boy taking a pee I delivered a suitable sermon. Quite apt really considering where we were. During the age old bout I looked up and saw a face trying to peer into the darkened room through one of the corridor windows. I realised that it was her boyfriend who was from another ward. I put one foot against the door to stop him entering the room. Gaynor bit her finger in order to stifle the scream that was gathering at the back of her throat like a Gulf of Mexico tornado waiting to unleash itself. The boyfriend tried the door but soon gave up assuming it to be locked. We both finished at the same time like a train hitting the buffers with no noise.

A short time after this I went to have a game of pool in the O.T. room. The boyfriend of Gaynor and a relative of his were engrossed in a game. I strolled over to them and asked if I could take on the winner. Without the old fashioned method of both armies arranging the kick-off time for a battle to commence, the relative hit me over the head with a cue. As they were raining blows on my semi-protected head my old friend adrenaline kicked in. Seconds later I thought I should have asked the rest of the people in the room if they wanted to take on the winner. Thank goodness at that moment in time there were no members of staff in the room. Fortunately, no one said anything so by the time the staff found the boyfriend and his relative groaning in one corner I was long gone.

I returned to my ward sat on the chair next to my bed. Time was spent thumbing through a magazine and becoming engrossed in one particular story. My solitude was broken by the sound of a young woman asking me if I had a cigarette to spare. I focussed on the speaker and recognised her as Linda from the ward above ours. My smile was met with a gleam in her eye and taking the plunge I asked her if she fancied going somewhere quiet. Continuing my immersion into an educational mode I took her up to the Seminar room. The thing that has always stuck in my mind was that after I had stood up I looked down at her and to my astonishment I realised that one of her stockings was brown and the other one was black. Even now I cannot say for sure whether she was plainly confused or that my medication was stronger than I thought. The fact that I left the room roaring with laughter put an end to what could have been an interesting interlude.

The Occupational Therapist asked everyone to state what their interests were. One of my main responses was swimming. This dovetailed very well with their programme of fitness and coordination. Before long, four of us were taken to the main leisure centre for an afternoon of swimming and general keep fit work. This suited me nicely as it was an all expenses paid activity and a break from the hospital. My swimming improved along with my general fitness. It is hard to understand that a breakdown is happening and it is harder to understand that recovery is taking place. I did not know for sure why I was still in the system. No one really explained anything to me and part of me did not want to ask. My feelings of loneliness and isolation were slowly passing along with the stigma that is associated with mental illness. As an example of the recovery that I was making the hospital agreed to allow my Grandmother to accompany me on a coach trip to Bridlington. This was one of her favourite seaside places and the happiness that we shared on that day has remained with me even though the exact details of the day have become blurred with the passing of time. One thing I do recall is taking her into a pub. The Cap'n would never have allowed her to go in a pub without his consent and she giggled like a sixteen year old. She was more nervous than the other fifty or so trippers from the hospital but could not help drinking more than the 'just the one glass' of milk stout. What a day.

The trip gave me quite a lift and I was feeling more like the old J until I went into the servery for breakfast a few days later. There was a long queue so I decided to have a smoke whilst the queue went down. I went over to ask a so called hard case for a light for my cigarette. His response, for reasons no one ever knew, was to throw a cup of scolding hot tea in my face. The pain I suffered coupled with the shock of it triggered a huge response from me. I grabbed hold of him and dragged him to the stair well. We exchanged punches all the way up to his ward where the staff eventually pulled me off him. Mark, the Charge Nurse from downstairs, coaxed me to the seclusion room. Once again, the liquid cosh was administrated to my system via the area that no man has the right to. Mark was the ultimate professional and I bore him no malice. The injection squad were a different kettle of fish. Their tactics were always the same. Mob handed and jab them quick with not so much as an excuse me.

My resentment at being jabbed again bubbled up like bile from an upset stomach. This was not the way it should be and I felt impotent in having my judgements of fairness being disregarded. So, the two days of solitary confinement in the seclusion room resulted in my internal barriers being shored up. Back on the ward my involvement with anybody or anything was at an all time low. One or two of the staff talked to me in a sympathetic manner but my head told me that they should be talking to the decision makers not me.

A scrap of a conversation between two of the younger staff discussing a local night club was overheard by me. That night, I took off to the said night club for an evening out and some fun. As a young man I wanted to join in teenagers pursuits and doing the night club scene was one of them. Due to the amount of alcohol I consumed coupled with my medication I became what is commonly known as 'well passed it'. Well pissed it was more like the case.

On my return to hospital at the ungodly hour of 3 a.m. in the morning, I was met with a posse of the largactil squad. They had arranged themselves down the corridor leading to the shower/bath area like the principles at an American wedding. The only trouble was that I was not exactly the blushing bride and they were not the bridesmaids. A leery, dog's breath member of staff ordered me to take a bath. In my innocence I said that I would have a shower in the morning. A firm insistence was the only response to my statement. "Get in the bath now", was growled the repeated order. The part of my brain that was functioning at a higher level rang a warning bell somewhere deep in my subconscious. If I undressed and had a bath the squad would have me at a disadvantage. My head dropped and I thought what the hell. I stepped into the bath/shower area and undressed. As I was climbing into the bath I became aware of the fact that female members of staff were standing there looking at me. If they had been as naked as me I don't suppose that I would have been bothered but in this instance my manly pride welled up. Even in my naked state I thought enough is enough. The Charge Nurse was the first person in my sights. Out of the bath I leapt and grabbed hold of the Charge Nurse's collar. I bent my knees and flipped him straight into the bath like a missionary baptising heathens in a river. No God bless though. The next member of staff made a lunge at me and he narrowly avoided being dunked like an apple in a barrel of water at a fun fair. An almighty kick off occurred and the staff went down so easily it was reminiscent of a bowler scoring a strike. The word went out and help was arriving from all quarters of the hospital. Even the porters joined in and it must have been strange for them as the only severe action they see is a frightened patient going off for an operation. There I was, in my glory, lashing out at whatever was moving in my vicinity. At one point, so I was told later, nine of the staff piled in and almost pinned me to the mattress in the seclusion room. With an ear piecing roar I reared up and moved the lot of them off me. Even in my angry state I became aware of police dogs barking. Apparently, the word had gone out and the boys in blue turned up expecting a full scale riot. The only thing they came across was a living Greek statue by the name of J.

No matter what, the fight cannot carry on with the boys in blue so I meekly gave in. Once again, the needle was rammed into my pin cushion of a body and the cosh was injected.

Later that morning, I woke up and I was immediately disorientated. My familiar surroundings were different and I was in a smaller ward. A member of the day staff trotted up to me and explained that during the night a female Psychiatrist had transferred me out of my usual ward. Over the following days, the doctor gave me a thorough examination and recommended a different course of medication and treatment. To every ones surprise my behaviour stabilised and I began to feel more assured and relaxed. I improved to such an extent that I was allocated my own room and asked if I would carry out simple duties in and around the ward.

In the next room to me was the hard case that I had fought up the stairs. He quickly acknowledged my status and decided early on that it was more advantageous to be my friend than my enemy. Before long, we were wheeling and dealing in cigarettes and anything else that turn a quick profit. No drugs though. The hospital was only too willing to whistle up the largactil squad for a spot of medical darts.

To make my room more homely I installed a television and some other personal items. My usual chat up line to any willing or soon to be converted girls was to invite them to watch a programme on television. "What programme is that?" enquired one pretty little thing. A nature programme was my reply.

The improvement in my general well being and mental state improved dramatically. This was all due to the excellent diagnosis of the doctor and the correct medication. If only I had been diagnosed correctly at an early stage the mishaps and reactions from me would never had happened. It is too easy to inject someone with largactil as a means of subduing them. Sometimes, it is harder to find out what the root causes are of a patient rather than relying on an overuse of strong tranquilisers. The conception namely the injection of drugs, as the only medical solution belongs, quite rightly, in the dustbin of medical thinking. It was also an important time for me as I could easily still be in the system receiving drugs at the whim of some outdated doctor. Interestingly enough, I have never been injected with largactil since the bath night.

My relationship with my new staff and fellow patients was at an all time high. My self esteem was raised due to my realisation that I was on a ward where the wearing of every day items of clothing was the norm and not pyjamas and slippers. The doctor, Dr. Prescott, advised me to join the 'back to work' group. This was a new initiative created by Bert Williams to rehabilitate patients and enable them to earn extra income. Through Bert's hard work a group of us set up a car wash area to clean the cars of staff or visitors to the hospital. The amount of extra income I received was not a large amount but it gave me control of my own weekly expenditure and a sense of ownership.

It was a fine summer's day when I marched off for my daily stint at the car wash. The paid member of staff supervising us was known to all and sundry as Uncle Ernest. He requested me to tidy up the hut where all the equipment was kept. To my utter delight a girl who worked with us was also given the same work detail. She was known to all as Shaky Sandy. This was due to the constant shaking she had caused by the recovery from alcohol abuse. I realised that we had a bit of time together so I started flirting with her. When I asked her if she was 'topped up' she replied that it had been a while since she had a fella. With that, I kissed her twice and responding to her eager movements spread her across the car wash sponges. We certainly lived up to our claim of done by hand. Shaky and I coupled up the hose pipe as and when we fancied it without ever being considered an item.

Chapter 14: Rehab Hostel

We still met at odd times when I was eventually discharged from the hospital and placed in a hostel designated for the rehabilitation of ex mental health patients. I was still a day patient at the hospital and every day I would attend the hospital and work on the car wash. During this time, I received visits from my Father and sister Marina. No one else came to see me due to a combination of a misplaced stigma and my conditioning as part of the hospital system. Perhaps, I was partly suffering from being institutionalised and I was slowly drifting from my roots. The people within the system were now my family and friends.

Within the hostel I was assigned my own room and quickly adapted the routine of the place. After breakfast I would catch a bus and report to the Day Ward at the hospital. After taking the prescribe dosage I would work on the car wash until it was time to go back to the hostel. Weekends found me strolling around Rotherham and keeping a low profile. My visits to the Cap'n were hit and miss but whenever I turned up they would greet me with the same love and warmth as always.

My Father had by this time opened up yet another gym for weight training and body building. He encouraged me to attend and I went along three times per week and often at weekends. By my nineteenth birthday I was bench pressing 300 lbs. weight and I realised that my body shape had altered dramatically. Soon, I was receiving admiring glances from the ladies and on some occasions I was the object of wolf whistles from the opposite sex. Bit by bit my self confidence returned as well as my mental strength.

The hostel was a huge place near Rotherham town centre. To gauge the size of the place it later became an old age person's home. The women had the upstairs rooms and the men were based on the ground floor. All in all there were 36 residents staying in the hostel. The facilities included a dining room, pool table and a communal television/ video room. The room consisted of a single bed, wardrobe and a couple of chest of drawers. Not exactly the Hilton but at least it was clean and tidy with a linen and towel change twice per week. The couple who ran the hostel had their own accommodation attached to the building. Their Son was called Ian and over a period of time I became good friends with him. Quite often, on video nights, he would obtain the storeroom keys and pass me bottles of pop and chocolate biscuits that I quickly hoarded in my room like a squirrel waiting for winter.

At night time, on a rotational basis, there were members of staff to look after us. One of the staff was an Irish colleen who took a shine to me. She would provide me supper and snacks on my return from my Father's gym. This was at a late stage of the evening when the other residents were in bed.

At the time, she was the nearest I had to a proper Mother and I remember her with great affection.

My relationship with my Father picked up tremendously during this time. We started making it a habit to go for the proverbial quick drink straight after training. At long last we had common ground and I for one was grateful for it. A spin off from this new Father/Son bonding was my Father's understanding and sympathies with a little problem that I had. I had met a girl called Wendy at the Rawmarsh Cricket Club one Friday night. At that time, this was regarded as an adult Slag Bin. The stumbling block was that every time she tried asking about my circumstances I had to side track her at every turn. Well, I could hardly tell her that I lived in a mental health hostel. What am I? The Freddie Kruger of Rotherham. Also, I was not exactly milking the font of endless resources and my pocket rarely jingled with money. My Father, bless him, used to bail me out as far as the folding money was concerned and with a few inventive stories I kept her well clear of my carry on and existence. As usual, being a woman, she began to question me more and more until the point where I refused to lie any more. So it was that the long kiss goodnight time came and she went.

I had nowhere to go so back in the hostel again listening to the unreasoned views of the residents. One night a guy called Stan the Man was making a cup of tea. The rumour was that Stan the Man was a hard nut and likely to kick off for any reason. He was supposed to have demolished any number of staff at the hospital and had caused havoc at the hostel on numerous occasions. I reached across him and told him that I would make my own cup of tea. He forced his slightly crooked arm across my chest and uttered a noise like a load of sloppy manure being delivered on a concrete drive. Reputations are just that. Bang. And there went another reputation. By this time most reputations were going and mine was coming. Sorry, arrived.

Life is all about irony and it has a nasty habit of appearing every so often. Up on the top floor of the hostel was a black haired girl sporting a chest that Dolly Parton would have paid a fortune for. The irony was that she was being fancied by the hard case who I had sorted out during my last stay in hospital. The one I knocked up the stairs. That was good enough reason for me to have a go at her. There is instant love and immediate lust. My lust for her was that fast that I did not have time for love. We were like a pair of rabbits on heat on Noah's Ark. As is the way of it, a member of staff eventually caught us out. Early one morning I found her in the launderette doing her smalls. She agreed to do my large and off we went for it. No sooner had I put my particular comfort in her machine than a member of staff came into the room and denounced us.

Chapter 15: The Lodge

The upshot of all this was that I was eventually offered a half way house that was in the grounds of the hospital. The half way house was known as the Lodge and I shared it with a guy called Clem. Not only was I in the Lodge but I was now on full benefit plus my reward money from the back to work group. To rub salt in the wound, as cheeky as you like, I used to walk over to the unit and have all my meals for free. "Are you still a patient J?" they asked. "Still attached to the hospital", I would reply. Hey Ho.

It was Easter when Clem and I laid claim to the Lodge and we stayed for the next six months. My average score for women invited back to the Lodge to view my Elvis Presley posters was a new one every two weeks. Not counting the returns, one-nighters and the ones gagging for it.

My family where more keen to visit me now that I was in the Lodge and Samantha would often pop round with her boyfriend Tony. He was a good bloke who sadly died of knife wounds at a later stage. She would do some cooking for me and at other times I would take them for a drink at the nearest village.

Dr. Prescott, who I was still seeing as an outpatient, invited me for a weeks camping as a reward for the work I was doing with the 'Back to Work' group. This was the first time I had been camping since the army cadets and the enjoyment that I had endeared myself to every body on camp. Dr. Prescott saw the benefits that the week had given me and followed up this week by asking if I would like to go to Flamborough Head, near Bridlington for another weeks camping. In a sense, this was the first proper holiday that I had ever had. To some, the East Coast is not high on their must visit list but to me it was as good as a world wide exploration. I cooked for the camp most mornings and I was only too eager to carry out any task that I was asked to do. I felt as if I was in the community again.

My feeling of well-being encouraged me to undertake more duties in and around the hospital. These I carried out to the best of my abilities and to my surprise I was awarded reward money for doing them. How better then to reward people with kindness and dignity instead of shooting unknown grams of whatever into them at a moments notice. The staff had treated me with respect and in turn my self esteem rose to a point where I felt the need to give a return.

My newfound friend was Colin who was attending as a day patient. He was a fellow confederate who was working on the back to work group. His main job was to carry out painting and decorating for ex-patients who needed some improvements to their property. Over the next few weeks we used to go for the quick fag together and eventually we were paired as a team. Typical of me that I quickly realised that a three day job done in two gave us a day off. Naturally, we started to go drinking in the town centre pubs. Little did I know that he had been referred to hospital for a drink related problem. Colin used to turn up to work spic and span and it came as some surprise to me that he needed a drink like I needed my grub.

Once or twice I would go back to his house for tea with him and his wife. It soon became the custom to stay over for the night and the feeling of being in a family environment was very strong. I had missed it more than I realised.

Chapter 16: 'Mind' Accommodation

Just as the autumn leaves were falling with some meaning, Taj, a nurse from the hospital, informed me that my time at the Lodge was nearing its end.

He took me to a house in the Masbrough area of Rotherham to assess the viability of it becoming my home. I instantly liked the house especially as it was fully furnished from top to bottom.

Naturally, I recruited Colin and Bert to help me with the emulsion of the house and other little decorating jobs that spread all over. Very soon, it was looking really homely and for the first time in a long time I had a feeling of ownership. After a couple of weeks, during which I acclimatised myself to the daily routine of washing, cooking, cleaning etc., I thought that it was about time that I christened the house in the usual way.

Friday night found me propped up at the bar in the infamous Grapes pub listening to the latest noises from the D-J. Within five minutes an oriental looking girl propositioned me by the name of Lauren. I looked at my watch and told her it was my bedtime. The taxi could not come quick enough for me and I could not come quick enough for her. What a bonk. Although it is true that you do not make love to oriental girls sideways on with Lauren I don't think it would have made any difference. A week later, a member of the famous Flower Estate family in Sheffield called Johnson gave Lauren and me a lift to her house. On the way back the boys in blue pulled the car. A policeman asked Derek what his name and address was. Obviously, being wanted by the communities best he gave a false name and address. As the name given did not match the police vehicle check we were invited to sample the delights of the hotel police station. I insisted that I did not know him and that I had thumbed a lift. In my naivety I was trying to defend Derek plus, I am not a grass. If I had said that I knew him they would have asked me what his real name was. As it was, Derek was singing the same tune as me and the boys in blue had no option but to terminate my residential stay. They kept Derek of course.

As is the way, the 'boys in blue' taxi service was not running so I had to walk all the way home. The trouble was that I was covered all over with love bites given to me by Lauren as a result of a very interesting bout of passion.

My next conquest was a girl called Paula. I met her one evening down town when I was out and about with my Cousin Tex. We had decided to give the Cresta's Nightclub a try and it did not take too long to pull Paula. As Tex pulled Paula's best friend we decided to go back to Paula's house. She had two kids but that did not deter me from my rightful path. Tex had marked my card as to the marital status of Paula and that her ex-husband had some reputation as a big hitter. I absorbed the warning but my lust was taking hold of me, and the thought of the chance of bedding Paula replaced any feeling of doubt as to whether I should bother. I went upstairs to the toilet and whilst I was washing my hands I heard an almighty crash. The ex-husband had burst into the house and he was roaring like a wounded bull. I calmly walked down the stairs and delivered a package faster than the Post office could ever do. Out he went and outside he went. That's that thought I. Needless to say I went back inside to see to Paula. I had not gone all that way to finish the night by hand. Just as I was pulling my trousers back on after the bedroom bout the ex-husband came back. This time he was tooled up and he was waving a baseball bat around like an upturned windmill. "I am going to get you", he shouted. "You b*****d". I hit him. Down he went again. As he was going down I said, "Do it don't say it".

The ex-husband never bothered me again and I had a good relationship with Paula. We were at it for about ten weeks and in the early New Year of 1984 we were as close as close could be. We were certainly close but only when we were together. My agenda was not her agenda. Good grief, she had more baggage than the carousal at Heathrow Terminal. I mentally put her on the back burner but she was beginning to take our relationship more seriously.

I had by this time given Paula a key to my house and the arrangement was that she would come over and cook my tea if I was out with the back to work group. Meanwhile, yours truly had picked up on a little blonde number called Suzanne. What a girl. We arranged to meet during times when I was not seeing Paula and this was fine until the fateful day when Suzanne and I were enjoying taking turns looking at the bedroom ceiling. We were so engrossed in this simple activity that I never heard Paula let herself into the house. She literally caught us in the act and before she had stopped her first scream the key had hit me on the head. Her next scream ended when she was outside and I never saw Paula again.

Suzanne was not too well pleased as I had told her that I was single guy. I managed to convince Suzanne that I had finished with Paula and that she was stalking me. See, before my time again.

Suzanne became my girl and we were very much the courting couple. We often went around the town pubs but always ended up in the commonly known pub The Zoo. One night, a gorilla came up to me by the name of Roy and told me to back off from Suzanne. He had half a lager in his hand for Suzanne and used his other hand to wave me away. As soon as Suzanne had taken the drink from him I gave him the lower Kimmy kiss. The jukebox began to play a record that had not been paid for. I realised that it was because the gorilla had fallen against the jukebox.

I realised that Suzanne had become too much hassle for me and I did not want to spend my time entertaining her by fighting with anybody who thought they had claim on her. Goodbye to Suzanne for now and off for another adventure.

Chapter 17: Year of the Miner's Strike

As the March winds were blowing litter around the main square in Rotherham, I literally bumped into a yet another blonde coloured haired woman. What a piece. Her shopping went everywhere and as a gentleman does, I helped to pick up the various bits. So, what's your name then, I asked her. She replied that her name was Janet. "O.K", said I. "So what do you want to drink then?" After a long cup of tea she asked me if I would help her with some more bits and pieces, as I was the perfect gentleman. She explained that she lived in the Broom area of Rotherham and that she was moving to another house in Dalton. Without further ado I went with her to the house in Broom and went in. Sitting on a settee was a guy watching television. He languidly looked over in my direction and carried on viewing his television programme. I just thought that this guy was a tenant in a shared house. It was much later when Janet and I were celebrating the first flush of lust in her new bed that night that she revealed that the guy was now her ex. What a start to what turned out to be a long relationship for me.

One of the early drawbacks to this coupling was the age difference. I was now nineteen and she was twenty-nine. When we went out to a pub I used to tell people that I was twenty-four. This state of affairs went on until our parting. It was much later that I found out that she had her suspicions that I was younger and that she used to knock at least five years off her true age when asked. White lies maybe, but age does not come into it when the bedroom light goes out.

Her job at the time was a Psychiatric Nurse at a hospital in Wakefield. What a turn around, an ex-service user giving the service a return.

Janet had two lovely daughters and they became a surrogate family in many ways. One of the odd things about going round to Janet's house was having a family meal at the dining table. The last time that I had had a family meal was when I was last at the Cap'n's deck. Soon, I was going to the house every day for at least one meal and afters. Being a nurse, she did not have a problem with the fact that I was still attending the hospital on a regular basis. The back to work programme was providing me with enough funds to take Janet out at least once per week and that seemed to be enough for her to share her duvet with me.

These were happy times for me, so when a local guy, called Bones from Masbrough, was thrown out of his flop I offered him the opportunity to stay at my house. Naturally, for two days I was over at Janet's doing what a man has to do. On the third day, my Father came to see me and told me that Bones was a drug addict. "How do you know? I asked him. "I know", was the enigmatic reply. "Get rid of him right now". So off we went to turf Bones out of the house. When we arrived I was furious to discover that there were about twelve guys in the house chasing the dragon. I chased them all right. Out of the house and out of the district. Bones was grovelling and whining when, quite unexpectedly, Big Bob turned up. "What's his problem then J?" As I was telling him, Big Bob dropped Bones in one. I dragged the crumbled form outside and shut the door. As I was cleaning up the house I kept coming across tin foil and traces of heroin on the table. I was relieved that the boys in blue had not turned up, as I would have been in the frame for aiding and abetting. On reflection, this was my first introduction to back street drugs. I was angry and intrigued at the same time.

I was in a bit of a mood by the time I returned to Janet's house. As I entered the kitchen, one of Janet's dogs, a red setter, walked into the room. The setter was on heat and was housebound for a while. In a mad two minutes, Janet's other dog, a Jack Russell, scampered into the kitchen and immediately locked himself in the charms of Amber. Needless to say, the pups were the oddest looking mongrels ever seen. The sight of Ben blazing away gave us a laugh. The laughter grew louder when Janet and I simultaneously looked at the dogs and then each other. The dogs were downstairs and we were upstairs.

One night, a local character called Cockney Rob called in on his way home from the pub. On the stove was a pan that was full of scrap meat being rendered down for the dog's next meal. Without any airs or graces Rob picked up a fork and stabbed a piece of the meat and started to eat it. I went from amicable to game on within seconds. He was knocked out of the house and deposited over the next door neighbour's wall. The bush telegraph soon drummed news of this encounter and the next thing I knew I was offered a job as a bouncer at the infamous Dalton Grapes pub. I reclined the offer as I thought that I had enough hassle in my life without throwing out some incapable reveller for having one too many. Besides, I had a reputation as a protector rather than as an enforcer.

My status with Janet's daughters was growing all the time and even now I look back with great fondness at the times we had and the closeness I felt towards them. I still come across Shelley and Debbie during my trips to Rotherham town centre and we always have good crack about the old days. We always honour Janet in our conversations as she sadly passed away in the late nineties.

Although Janet figured predominately in my mind, that part of me that was a man began to look in other places. What started off as the usual checking out of a woman, as men tend to do, slowly accelerated to a point where my lower brains began to move from fantasy to reality. One day, Janet's eldest daughter gave me some weenie grief and the conversation did not go particularly well. Janet, naturally, defended her daughter so I left the house in the puzzled way that most men do when women give them the verbals and the man asks himself the question, 'What the hell'. My teatime walkabout ended with me arriving back at Masbrough and I entered my house with a heavy heart. Just as I put the kettle on for a cup of tea my sister Samantha breezed in complete with her trademark grin and conspiratorial look. "Guess who has just moved in near me", she opened her conversation. 'No idea', I replied. She began to explain that Shana had moved in from South Kirby near Barnsley. 'What is she like then?' was my immediate response. Samantha suggested that I went up there and find out for myself. So, I called in at the Cap'n's house for permission to come aboard and drink his typhoon rum. Of course, when I left, it just happened that my journey home was via Samantha's place; or more to point, Shana's. A few minutes later I knocked on Shana's door and this brunette with a large pair of melons answered the door. "Hello, I'm J". "Yes", she said. "I have had the full dossier on you". "If you have, then you will be coming out with me". She giggled and said "Yes".

A couple of days later on my twentieth birthday I escorted Shana to the Champs Nightclub that was fixed next to the Grapes pub at Dalton. This was rubbing salt in the wound, as this was the drinker that I usually took Janet to. This was certainly a case of regrets as I choose to stay with Shana rather than Janet. Janet did not deserve this betrayal and I have always had some misgivings when I think of her and those days. Needless to say, Shana and I went back to the love nest known as my house and when I said come here my princess she went wild. I was soon on and off with her more than the passengers going on and off a bus. She very quickly was blessed with the nickname of Landlady as there was more traffic going through her house than a lorry driver's bed and breakfast place.

During one of my on periods with her I took her downtown to a bar, sometimes nightclub. Soon, we were joined with our Samantha and her latest bloke. Samantha was seven months pregnant at the time and this was a rare night for her. Her man, who fortunately was too small to do any real damage, decided it would be a good idea to tell a bouncer to join the rest of the penguins in the zoo. He was asked, in the way that bouncers do, to leave the premises. In the skirmish that followed Samantha was pushed to one side and cried out with some degree of pain. My brain said Family, hurt, defend and then the adrenaline rushed in. Quite simply, I went berserk. The bouncer, who had hold of Samantha's bloke, registered one brief flash of pain before falling unconscious after my well delivered head butt. The other bouncers came rushing towards me like the Zulus at Rorke's Drift and they dropped as readily as the Zulus in that famous battle. After the ball was over I coolly sat down and brushed off imaginary bits of dust off my coat. A few minutes later I motioned my party to leave and I strutted out with my head going like a prize cockerel pecking for corn.

The fight is still mentioned today during reminisces by those who were there.

My Cousin Tex was knocking a woman off that I had the hots for. We went as a foursome once every so often and all that ever did for me was to make me want her even more. One night, I was round at the Landlady's house having some late supper when Tex and his lady walked in. Later, I went to bed with the Landlady and Tex and his lady climbed into the same bed. Without further ado I turned his lady onto her back and went at it all guns blazing for ten minutes. I only stopped when my left ear could not take the noise of her screaming anymore. I looked over at Tex and he was on his back with the Landlady on the top of him like some cowgirl riding the bucking bronco. All I concentrated on was the sight of the Landlady's finest bouncing around like two wild ferrets having a fight to the death. At long last the Kentucky Derby came to an end and we all staggered downstairs for a drink and a rest. All of a sudden, the Landlady slapped Tex's lady across the face and called her a dirty bitch. It later transpired that she regretted the incident and was full of remorse for herself. No surprise then that she ordered Tex and I out of her house like an angry drill sergeant on the parade ground. 'And you two can f*** off as well', came the sound of her voice as Tex and I, an arm around each other's shoulder, were laughing that much that we could not walk in a straight line.

Tex began to stay over with me at Masbrough more and more and we became very close again. We seemed to have more women than hot dinners and we dropped into the habit of addressing every female in the house as pet. It was only because we had given up trying to remember anybody's name and this seemed the easiest thing to do.

Ours was an oasis of 'who bonks who cares'. One night, there was a knock at the door and this guy was standing there breathing like a raging bull. Is that twat of a Cousin of yours f****** my woman? 'Tex', I shouted, 'There is someone here for you'. Tex got up out of bed and came downstairs with just his trousers on. He went straight outside and dropped the raging bull quicker than a prostitute's knickers. He turned round and went back upstairs to finish his conquest.

Soon, it was the festive season's and parties where being arranged and gatherings sorted. I was invited to the New Year's Eve party at a house over in Meadowbank. My escort for the evening was none other than the Landlady. This was only due to the fact that she was in the same pub as me before the party. We arrived at the party swimming in good spirits and launched into the swing of things with a great deal of enthusiasm. Shana went to the bathroom and I became aware that she had been gone for quite a while. I decided to investigate and I stumbled across some guy determined to end the year with a bang with the Landlady. I hauled him off her to a sound similar to someone pulling his or her foot out of wet mud. He saw the traditional fireworks before the official ones where set off. The next thing I knew I was fighting four of them at the same time. It was like a scene out of the Three Musketeers except it was all for one and bugger the rest. The fight went out into the street and I could swear that I trampled over every garden in the street. Bodies littered the road like a tramps benevolent party and I was still throwing punches like a bowler at a game of rounder's. Even in those days there were grasses and before long the boys in blue arrived to their clarion call of pulsing sirens. I was covered in blood and when the first policeman approached me I muttered something about a riot and look what they did to me. It was not long before I was sent to the hospital to be fixed up. Bit by bit the waiting area filled up with bodies that I had hit or frightened silly. Happy New Year.

Chapter 18: Happy New Year

New Year's Day saw Samantha and me wandering down the street slightly worse for wear back to the party. Not so much for the hair of the dog but more a case of full mop of the horse. Samantha was nearly full term now and the sight of her wobbling along in that peculiar gait that only pregnant women can muster brought me to my knees in laughter. "Weebles can wobble but they can't fall over", was all I could sing between tears. Cheers to you and happy New Year was my toast to Samantha.

I entered the house and eventually went into the lounge. The husband of the house was sitting in an armchair with his nose pointing 180 degrees to the norm. What a sight. "When are you joining the circus?" I asked. He looked at me and said the inevitable make up line of, "We want no more trouble". With that, I said cheers and poured another drink down my throat. Yes, I know, my stomach rumbles regular but it also becomes thirsty. The day passed peacefully and all agreed that this was better than grassing to the police and having the boys in blue sniffing around everyone's business.

Towards the end of January, Tex and I met up with the Swallow sisters. We had known them for a while and we decided to ask them out for the proverbial drink, chat and back to bed. Back at my house in Masbrough we had another drink before the evening keep fit session. One of the girls suddenly suggested that we all smoked a spliff. This was a new one on me and, before my fears of seeing ants crawling up the wall took hold, the youngest sister said that it would relax us and put us in the mood. Enough said, thought I. Phew! What a kick in, that was. It certainly put me in the mood and it certainly made me put the mood in. So, my first introduction to smoking marijuana was quite an event.

It did not take long for me to adopt the spliff smoking mentality and I would go to the pubs that mattered to buy a wedge. This went on for three months and yet again I was on the prowl for a marijuana joint. I went into one of my usual haunts and asked the supplier for some stuff. To my annoyance he said that he was completely out of grass and the only thing that he had was heroin. No chance, I thought. Dealers always try this tactic and I was not prepared to go down this route. So, I went for a drink in another pub and I was standing at the bar sipping my pint contemplating the world and my navel. Further down the bar were two guys from my old estate. They sidled up to me and asked me if I knew anybody who wanted to buy a video recorder. I thought that I would ask a couple of people in the pub if they were interested. One of the guys I asked in the pub was going out with one of my Cousins. He said no but he could do me an ounce of amphetamine sulphate (speed). I went back to the two Muppets at the bar and put this deal to them. They immediately said that they were interested in the deal. One of them said that they would give me twenty pounds if we could carry out the deal at my house. Easy money I thought so I went along with the proposals. Later on, the deal was done and my Cousin's fellah went on his way. The two Muppets were still hanging about the house and they asked me if they could try the speed there. Minutes later they were on a high and they pressured me to try some. Eventually I gave into their coaxing and I was injected by the older of the two who was called Trippy Dave (for obvious reasons). A rush went straight through my body, similar to a thundering orgasm.

To my shame I have to say it was exhilarating at the time. Of course, little did I realise the damage this regression had caused. I had spent so long turning the corner only to give in so easily on a whim. Thus began a champagne lifestyle on a sherbet income. For nearly two years I drifted in and out of a chemical world. The magic carpet ride was to end when love visited me but more of that later.

The speed scene was known by its more usual term of "the whizz scene". There were always plenty of good looking girls prepared to dabble in drugs and I had dabbled with them too. If I seem a bit vague about this period of my life it is because I was not proud of my involvement and I would sooner forget it. I am escaping my dues by not relating events and stories but quite a few people who were experimenting in those days lead a respectable life now and I am thinking of them as I write.

One event I will recall with some clarity was my pilgrimage to the Reading festival. I went down with Trippy Dave and a couple of his associates. We soon pitched our tent and blended in with the other festival goers. I placed some green electricians tape around my wrist and went through the gates in the middle of a bunch of hyperactive girls. Although the band that was main heading the festival was not one that I cared for I really enjoyed the crack. A combination of drink and selected sweeties enhanced the enjoyment of being at the festival. Odd, though, that I managed to have a fabulous weekend that included no sexual activity.

On my return home I dragged myself in my house and slumped in my armchair. The next thing that I knew there was a banging on my door. Trippy Dave was at the door and he asked me to open the boot of my mate's car. I opened the boot and to my astonishment it was like looking in Aladdin's cave. The boot was full of stolen gear including a bag of speed. "What the hell is all this lot then?" I asked. It turned out that, unbeknown to me, the Rotherham contingent had been out and about in Reading shoplifting everything and anything. They had used my mate's car as the bank for their stolen loot. For once, I was squeaky clean without a blemish on my virgin white character.

My life became like a leaky colander. It was full of holes with the occasional oasis of reality and clear memory showing through. Odd things come to mind but not necessarily in the order that they occurred. One such event was the day when I went out on the beer as an alternative to the drugs. I met up with one of Canklows (a notable area of Rotherham) residents nicknamed nuts and bolts. He was called such because, allegedly, his teeth were missing or jagged as if he had been chewing nuts and bolts. We went in the now defunct Polish Club, as it was one of the few places where a thirsty man could assuage his urge in the days before all day drinking. Naturally, I proceeded to salute the world, my mates and my stomach. I was in the smaller room having a game of pool and minding my own business. In walked nuts and bolts followed by a couple of washers who were the wrong size to begin with. Nuts and bolts had a fierce some reputation around Rotherham and, even though the Polish Club contained, as it would, quite a few notables, everyone lowered their heads and pretended to be interested in their bootlaces. He went into the larger room and started offering everyone out. People shrank back from him. This was partly due to his reputation and mostly to his dog's breath. I hit the pool table with my hand in despair. It would only be a matter of time before his instant weed killer escaped from his mouth followed by his habitual spit. NNNUUUURRRR. He went. Like a cow with terminal constipation. "It's the Boston Strangler". He always called me this because he once accused me of attempting to throttle a mate of his in Boston Park, Rotherham. A right load of tosh but we are talking about nuts and bolts here. I had two choices. Knock him out with my right hand or my left hand. The right hand went first and missed by a gnat's left testicle. Someone said later that they felt the wind rush past them from the blow and they were in the toilets. I spun round and caught him a left hook that Henry Cooper would have dined out on for years. The paramedics were soon on the scene and it was a surprise to most people there that the undertakers were not called first. A dose of smelling salts, familiar to him in many guises, eventually brought him round. He spat out enough bits of teeth to make a cannibals necklace. My reputation was finally cemented as surely as nuts and bolts demise. In the next three weeks three other people went up against him and showed him the way home. You see, I am not and never have been a bully. That guy did nothing socially, only intimidate or extort people for fun.

That was the last time I was ever wary of any foe. It does not mean that I don't underestimate anybody but the fear of losing is not a consideration. If anyone beats me now it is only my shadow they are defeating, not the real J.

Another patch of memory was my twenty-first birthday celebration in the Cresta's Night Club. I was flying high and so was the inevitable blonde piece called Dawn who I was dancing with. Before long, she invited me back to her flat to end my birthday day with a bang. It was only when I started looking at the photographs on the side table that I realised that she was the girlfriend of Speedy Steve. Speedy was having a residential holiday courtesy of H.M.P.S. She asked me if I wanted to stroke her pussy. I turned round and she was sitting on a chair fondling her cat. Not me.

I have never been with a mate's girlfriend or partner and never intend to.

Christmas of that year started off rather dismally. I had recently left my house at Masbrough to take up residence in a flat at Kimberworth Park. I had not had enough time to decorate or furnish the place as I wanted. At eight O'clock on Christmas Eve I went round to the Cap'n's house for a glass of something and to wish them well for Christmas. They went to bed at nine thirty as usual and I trudged back to my flat feeling more and more despondent and lonely. I lay on my bed and no sooner had I done so when there was a knocking at the door. Who else but Speedy Steve. "What the hell are you doing here?" I asked. Taking you to the party at Splodge's flat. "Need you ask", I said, and off we went to the Party. Friends in lots of respects at the time but on reflection it was a sad time hanging around with drug associates.

New Year's Eve found me running round all over the borough looking for amphetamines. I was suffering from a dose of Cold Turkey and I did not fancy spending such an important night on a downer. My travels took me as far as Sheffield to a dealer's place known as Pop. One of my fellow travellers was a junky known as the Doc. He was called this because his chief claim to fame was that he could find any vein in the human body in pitch black conditions. Pop sorted us out with some chemical or other. We immediately loaded up and wished each other a happy New Year. Such optimism then sounds, and is, the true falsity of all time. How many of the users from those days are still wishing people happy New Year now? I have been to eight drug related funerals from the time of my first intake. Having 'sadly missed' put on my gravestone by some over-rich dealer is not my intention.

The best part of the New Year was spent either on a cloud or shivering under my blankets after a bad hit. Days, even weeks, passed me by with no permanent memories lodging in my mind.

I do remember, though, the night I took Suzanne back to her flat. She had just received the keys for it and there was absolutely nothing in it. The lights did not work, as the meter had not been switched on. That meant no heating and it was freezing in there. I was wearing an army coat for warmth and being the gentleman I am I took off my coat and offered it to Suzanne. She laid it on the floor and laid down on it. I only gave it to her to keep her warm but she obviously thought that physical exercise would do the trick. I certainly gave her another one, or was it two or three? Shortly after that I put her on a National Express coach to Aberdeen. She was off for three weeks to visit her sister who was in the Shetland Isles. The next time I saw her was eight years later with five kids in tow.

Chapter 19: The Grapes Bust

The Grapes Bust was destined to go down in the history of Rotherham and especially the East End of the borough as the bust of the century. The Grapes pub contained more drug dealers per area of seating than Columbia on a good day. It was said that you only had to stand at the bar ordering a pint of beer and breathe in to get high. The slogan over the door was, 'we have it, what do you want?'. When the Small Faces sing the lyrics 'What do you do there, I get high' I still think of that place. One evening, I was in a car with three mates and Geraldine was driving. We decided to call in the Grapes for a few supplies before heading up to town for a night out. Oddly enough, I remained in the car and told the rest of the crew that I did not want anything. I was seeing a girl that night and I did not want my performance to be less than fabulous. They came out of the pub and climbed into the car in a giddy state. No sooner had we travelled a few hundred metres than I spotted the boys in blue transport machine. "Drugs squad", I instinctively yelled out. I told the other three to put whatever they were carrying in their mouths and hope for the best. By the time the lead pointy hat tapped on the window of the car the other three were chewing for England. He accused us of having drugs and ordered us out of the car. Political correctness had somehow blown passed Rotherham and we were treated to an old fashioned 'hello, hello, hello, what's this 'ere'. Whilst the lead boy in blue was asking Geraldine for her driving licence a group of plain clothes policemen jumped out of their hiding place and surrounded us. "We are the drugs squad", said one of the donkey coat wearing brethren, "And you're nicked". One of my mates said, 'I f****** knew it'. A quick nod of the head and a stainless steel paddy wagon came roaring up to us and we were politely asked to get on board for a mystery charabanc trip. They gave us a cursory pat down and off we jolly went.

The paddy wagon stopped before long and we were herded out like cattle at the stockyards on a cold Chicago day. Into the station we went and not for a single ticket. We were escorted to a large room that was full of pointy hats and druggies. Everybody was standing there muttering obscenities and complaining about anything and everything. The police kept coming in and moving out three or four people at a time for a full strip search. My turn came and I shuffled out with a couple of known faces. Whilst I was standing at the custody desk giving my inside leg measurement and the brand of knickers that my Grandma wears, a young pointy hat trainee came in with a spotty faced youth who made a sick parrot look well. It was obvious from the stares of everybody concerned that these two guys were in the wrong place at the wrong time. I was facing the custody desk and behind me were the cells where the strip searches were taking place. The memory of the time in hospital came flooding back and I was determined that I would not be forcibly searched.

As the spotty faced youth approached me I stood to one side and he was immediately whisked into the search cell. The cell erupted with laughter as the police realised that this guy should not have been stripped searched. In the confusion someone said to me that it was my turn. "Oh no", said I, "I have already been searched". Without further ado I was hauled off to a holding cell.

Apparently, this was a huge bust and involved more police than you see at the Christmas Ball. It was, I think, called Operation Rupert Bear. Not my bear bum though. They had turned the Grapes pub over and the cells were full of every known dealer, user, or vaguely interested. The police were determined to break the Grapes and its associated drugs tag once and for all.

Me, Tigger and The Doc ended up in the same cell. The next thing we knew was the door was pushed open and the spotty faced youth was hurtled in. He was on an all time grouse. Boy, was he mad. "You know what them bastards have just done?" he said, "They have just looked up my bleeding arse for a stolen motor bike". I would not have missed that night for the world. The laughter went on and on and on.

Eventually, the gallant three were escorted to the door and we gave our thanks for the bed and breakfast. "No tip mind", said Tigger. We set off for the town centre like Dorothy skipping down the yellow brick road.

The Grapes bust certainly cleared the Grapes pub out and very little drug activity went on there after the event. No surprise then, as mentioned, the Grapes pub has been razed to the ground and is now just a car lot before its next reincarnation.

The last time that I ever went in the Grapes was when I went to see my Cousin Tex. I had not seen Tex for a while and he was going out with a woman called Molly. Within minutes of being in the place Tex and Molly kicked off with a huge row. I decided to calm Tex down by asking him to leave the pub and come back to my flat. We were heading towards the door when two Scottish guys, left over from a Scotland versus England match, started on me. They were telling me to mind my own business. In a polite way I explained that Tex was my Cousin and I was stopping him from getting into trouble. The problem was that the Scottish duo was not in a mood for listening and they were determined to run their own agenda. They caught up with me in the car park, or should I say early bottle bank, and started a fracas. It has always been apparent to me that if they come in a pair then they can't be much good. It did not take long before I hurdled one of them to one side. I should have been in the Highland games tossing the caber judging by the way I removed him from the fight. The other one met his Bannock Burn with one hit. Not long after, the same two guys were in attendance at my Father's gym and they told him that I was the hardest bloke that they had encountered. I thought that was flattering, especially as I was smoking a fag with the other hand.

190

Chapter 20: Summer '86

The summer months were spent dabbling with a bit of whizz, a few women and my beloved Northern Soul. Sex, Drugs and Northern Soul. Not original but that was my life during the halcyon days of 1986. My choice of mates at the time was drawn from the drugs scene such as it was in sunny Rotherham. One lad who I mixed with on a frequent basis was a guy named Dunc. One night, I met up with him at the Cresta's night club. By the end of the night he looked absolutely out of it so I suggested that he left his car in Rotherham and that we caught a taxi back to his place. We bundled ourselves into a taxi and he mumbled the directions to the taxi driver and off we went. To my puzzlement we ended up at a house that I did not recognise. "Come on J", he yelled out, "If you are as good as they say you are you will be up in here". Odd choice of words, thought I, and it was not until we went into the house that I understood why he said it. Waiting for us were two delightful little fillies sitting on a settee grinning like Cheshire cats. What a night, or should I say weekend. It was early Monday morning when we left and could we hell as like walk in a straight line. The weekend was called a door key session. In other words, we would swap bedrooms and lock the door. The changeovers were happening so fast I never did find out who was who and who they were. When Dunc and I were wending our way back to Rotherham for his car I asked him for the names of the girls. "Does it matter?" he replied. Yes, I told him, for my little red book. "What book is that then?" he asked. I tapped the side of my head and said "My red book in here". Never forget a name or an address.

Tony G, one of the lads off the East Dene estate, always used to refer to me as the milkman. He reckoned that I had a larger round than a milkman in terms of women. The reason why I mentioned this is due to the fact that I was becoming more and more disillusioned with the drug scene. There were a lot of women on the scene and my attention was turning more to them than the drugs. However, some of the women used to offer bed and breakfast for drugs but I never paid for my enjoyment in that manner. The amount of drug intake was decreasing but there was still the perceived comradeship connected to the drug scene and I was not sure which direction to take or how to seek help for myself. Self denial is a strong motivator not to seek outside help or professional help. I knew that I was not advancing my life but somewhere, somehow, I had the belief that a light would shine and illuminate the path I should take.

My family were still giving me a huge amount of support, care and counselling. They would frequently seek me out for a chat or to bring me little treats like a packet of biscuits or things for the flat. Much as they tried I was still rejecting their overtures. Doing drugs is one thing, to admit taking drugs to close relatives is another. The self denial aspect is always there and despite the longing for drugs it prevents someone from opening their hearts and asking for help.

One of the side effects of drug taking is that a person is not always in full control of their judgemental capacities. As a consequence of using drugs I was eventually arrested by the police and finally sentenced to eighty community hours. Even though I have had this glitch this was the only time that I have faced the courts and been given a documented record.

I was trying to adapt an alternative lifestyle but the people on the drugs scene kept offering me freebies. Partly due to the fact that a druggie still prefers company of some sort preferably like minded people. Despite being a drug taker I was still a big lad and people doing deals needed me around as some form of protection. This was not what I wanted to do and I was forever racking my brains as to how I could distance myself from these associates.

I was taking stock of myself and little by little I started to realise that my former friends had moved on and that I was standing still at a fast pace. They were holding down steady jobs and one by one they were marrying their girlfriends and settling down. More and more of my time was spent wandering around the Rotherham club scene catching up on old friends and what was happening in their lives. One of my old mates invited me to a new nightclub that had been opened for a while and oddly enough I had never been in it. As it was near to my birthday I accepted the invitation. Sure enough, I turned up to the agreed meeting place and soon fell in with the crack and humour of my mates. Before long, we went into the nightclub and arranged our needed seating plans.

The night was going well and quite a few faces appeared in front of me to give their regards and to have a little chat. The feeling of belonging was beginning to warm me and I felt a sense of normality that I had not had for long enough. That was until Pat the Rat sauntered up to me with of all things The Landlady in tow. She was draped on his arm like an inexpensive hooker on the arm of a two bob millionaire. "She's with me now, Tuney", he belched at me with a sneer on his face. "So what? I replied, "I was there first and I am certainly not going to follow you". Even in his torpor state a flicker of intelligence flashed in his eyes as he slowly digested what I had said to him. Apparently, he had been knocking a few over like skittles in a back street pub and he had gained an inflated reputation for being a handy bloke. He swayed back on his feet and suddenly he whacked me one in the mouth. Normally I am not caught out like that but he looked such a washed up wreck I never thought for one minute that he would be so disrespectful. "Is that all you've got?" I asked him. As his brain was digesting what I asked him and whirling away trying to formulate a string of recognisable words that would make some sense to someone on his mental level I sent across the Lower Kimberworth hammer. He crashed between a chair and a table in one almighty thud. The excitement of it all was enough to make me go to the toilet to pass a comment on the attributes of Pat the Rat. I was just tidying up when in walked one of Pat the Rat's Muppets and head butted me. As luck would have it a doorman was standing at the toilet entrance watching proceedings. I immediately yelled out to the doorman, "You saw that". He immediately replied, "Get on with it". The Muppet stood there in a total blank wonderment at us two having a conversation after he had delivered what he thought was his best shot. With that I despatched him to a temporary world of shooting stars and loud almost musical noises in his head. Two in two minutes. Rock on J. Tune.

Here's me trying to ease up on things and the first time I go to a reputable night club this happens. The sequel to all this was that my Cousin Tex was waiting in the taxi rank outside when someone rushed up to him and told him that the toilet Muppet had head butted me. They failed to tell him that I had already taken him out and that he was standing outside trying to clear the incessant ringing in his head. Tex went straight across to him and decked him as a matter of principle. Not many in Rotherham can say that they were decked by two Tunes in the same night. To finish the night off a bouncer came out saw what happened and decided to have a go at Tex. That coincided with the arrival of J. Tune. Naturally, I leapt in to defend Tex. One crack later and the night club were advertising for new hired help. It took hours between the laughter, disbelief and complete enjoyment for us to piece together the sequence of events. Good job that CCTV was in its infancy and therefore no record of the events were recorded for prosperity. Could have been good on the programme a Question of Sport where they ask 'and what happens next'.

So, what does happen next? Well, in the aftermath of this escapade I decided to keep a low profile but still keep up my pecker with the ladies. Nearing Christmas, I went out with my mate Gank, one Saturday afternoon, to a notorious town centre pub named The Turf. Anybody who was anybody used The Turf at some point on their walkabouts. In the middle of the crowd the vision of my life appeared. She was strawberry blonde, legs, petite and the eyes to go. The grin was instantly switched on and off I went panting like a lap dog on heat. I asked her name and she told me that her name was Sadie. Her friend was called Yvonne but I already met her before. All four of us decided to go to the Polish Club for a few after hours drinks. Later, we went to Sadie's flat for a bite to eat and to continue the crack. We chatted for quite a while and eventually said our goodbyes. I was under the impression that Sadie did not care for me that much and I left it at that. The following day Gank and I went to the Eastwood pub for the Sunday lunch time session. To our delight Sadie and Yvonne were sitting there nursing a couple of small lagers. Naturally, we went across to them and had a chat for an hour or two. On leaving, Yvonne told me that she had a flat at Meadowbank and I told her that was my old stamping ground. She said that I could pop in for a cup of tea whenever I was passing there. So, one day, I went round to see her and helped her to move some rubbish and builders rubble. During the conversation Sadie was mentioned and Yvonne told me that Sadie was very interested in me and that she was up for a date if I wanted one. I left Yvonne the address of my flat and thought no more about it. One tea time, after work, Sadie knocked on the door of my flat and I could not believe my luck.

The moment that Sadie knocked on my door was the moment that I kicked drugs out of my door. My flat was not exactly overburdened with furniture so Sadie and I settled down on a large bean bag and we spent ages just looking at one another and shyly smiling as we attempted to say the things that were on our minds. Struggling to phrase the precise string of thoughts that were rattling around in my mind I blurted out that I was falling for her and that I could not help myself. At the same time, though, I told her that she would eventually break my heart. She said that she thought and felt the same things and that she would never hurt me.

Sadie stayed over at my place in all innocence and all we did was talk. Such was the respect that I had for her along with the feelings and emotions that were coursing through me. For the first time for a long time I felt that this time it was returnable. J-J was now a distant memory in terms of emotions and, dare I admit, love

Chapter 21: For the Love of a Woman

During the first flush of love or should I say lust (well, I am a Rotheramite and that's the way it is up here) I somehow kept my respectability and honour. For the first few weeks or so I used to sleep over at Sadie's place but I spent my nights in a single bed in a spare corner. Platonic love meets total respect that moved onto a burning desire in at a rapid speed. What on earth was happening to me? I spruced up considerably. An expensive haircut was followed by a visit to notable designer shops touched off with renewed efforts in the gym. Drug dealers began calling at my flat for business only to be told to F*** O*** in no uncertain terms. People from the drug scene were being put on the back burner and I began the process of annexing my ties with my previous associates. Time spent with Sadie was great time and I never felt like leaving her even if it was to go to the local shop for a packet of smokes.

We were officially an item from Boxing Day onwards. We had celebrated Christmas in grand style and we had ended up back at her place with love on our minds and a bottle of wine to kill the minutes between expressions of our love. Sadie had a week off work in the New Year and naturally I arrived at her place with not so much an overnight bag but a moveable wardrobe. John Lennon and Yoko Ono had already done the week in bed protest so we decided to do a Jason and Sadie week in bed non-protest. What was there to protest about? Any bloke who is capable would spend a week in bed with a woman. My bonus was that I was with a beautiful woman who I adored.

You may remember that I was given eighty community hours for my aberration. Naturally, as one would, I avoided the hours and pretended that I was not involved in that carry on. Being with Sadie pricked my conscience to such an extent that I asked to complete the set hours. The work involved me going with a gang of men to re-decorate the insides of selected churches. I eventually completed the number of hours required and it led me to think that if I could work for nothing in this gang I could work for someone and earn money. Not only that, Sadie had a paid job and I wanted desperately to provide some funds for our well being.

My sister Marina was courting an Italian guy who worked for a national chain of Pizza outlets. We quite often used to dine there in a foursome and it was a delight to me to be with a member of my family and my lady.

My euphoria with Sadie came juddering to a halt early in February when news came that the Cap'n's number one had died. I was heartbroken that my Grandmother had passed away. The shock I felt was over whelming and I was inconsolable. After all, this was the woman who had raised me and who had always given me love first before even asking how I was. She died on Valentines Day and it is rather fitting that such a woman with so much love for everyone else should die on the day celebrated for love.

Around this time Big Bob and I went on the knocker looking for work. On the knocker meant knocking on the doors of factories pleading for work. We eventually obtained a job in the industrial dismantling game. My duties were to dismantle an old steel works and to use burning equipment to cut through metal girders. Hard work and very dirty but it meant that I was earning a crust and more importantly earning pride. The money that I was earning improved my standard of life and I could go out at night knowing that I had worked for the right to spend my cash. My brother Dave split up with his partner and had being staying in some flops around the place. I offered him the opportunity to stay at my place as I was predominantly staying with Sadie.

My life became that of suburban bliss. There were weekly visits to the launderette, emptying the rubbish and taking Sadie her breakfast in bed on a Sunday morning. I was quite an all rounder really. No wonder her Mother Anita gave me the seal of approval. We still went to The Turf Tavern to see our friends and to make arrangements for couples only nights out. At long, long last I felt wanted for the right reasons and not for what I could dish out in terms of money or physical brawn. Everyone we met who I had not seen for a while always remarked how well I looked. I had put on a few welcome pounds thanks to Sadie's cooking and the climb down from the drug taking had helped to put colour back in my face. It was only a chance comment by someone to Sadie that made me realise that I was spending most nights with a grin on my face.

My defence of Sadie's honour was tested one day when the boyfriend of the girl next door banged on the door of Sadie's flat with some force. Apparently, there was a dispute with Sadie and this girl over a misplaced watch and blame and counter blame was on the agenda for days. I opened the door and faced down this anger filled Muppet who was frothing at the mouth on the doorstep. "What do you want first?" I asked him, "My knee, my head, my feet or this?" At that I hit him once and it was goodnight Vienna. Hence to say, we had no more knocks on the door. I was protecting my little flower, enough said.

During the summer, we went on days out to the seaside and to other tourist locations. Her Father Roy helped us to decorate her flat and bit by bit the quality of our surroundings was improved. Finally, on Remembrance Day (also her birthday), Sadie and I were engaged. I had been working Saturday mornings to pay for the engagement ring. It was a blue Sapphire set on a gold ring. It matched her habitual blue eye makeup. The date was set for the wedding and this was announced at the engagement party held at her Mother's house. One of my invited guests was none other than Gasping Gaz. He crashed out for the night on Sadie's Mother's settee and later threw the hospitality given to him back in people's faces. He was not on my original invitation list but Big Bob had pleaded the case for him and I had given in to

Big Bob against my inner beliefs. I was later to be proved right.

On the seventeenth of November, the year of our Lord, 1987 the Cap'n went to his own variety of Davy Jones Locker. I received the news whilst I was at work and I went straight to the Cap'n's ship. The pain that my soul was suffering was almost unbearable and I had great difficulty in stopping the willing tears that wanted to flow. He obviously had given up the will to live after the death of his life long soul mate. The loss of two such leading figures in my life was torment of the worst kind. I remember that I felt like passing out at frequent times and I really did feel physically sick to the bottom of my boots. They were in effect the parents that in some other time and place I would have had. It gives me a sense of pride knowing that wherever they are now if they read my heart they will see my love for them. In turn, I am sure if they could send me a message they would tell me not to be down for them but to rejoice in sharing their lives. Everybody has his or her time and so it was.

The funeral was held in Saint Thomas's Church, Kimberworth. The church was overflowing with family and friends. As an acknowledgement to the Cap'n we sang 'The Lord is my Shepherd' and his particular favourite, 'Jerusalem'. By the singing of the second verse there were many broken notes and sharp intakes of sobs. I held it together, on parade. This was my final tribute to the Cap'n and

I was determined to send the gallant old boy off with full colours.

During the informal wake family jokes concerning the Cap'n and anecdotes were in full flow. My favourite was the one concerning the Cap'n's older brother Joe who was a real hard case in his time. Apparently, one Sunday on church parade in jail, the roving Reverend stood up and in the shrill voice that back to front collar wearers have, said," Let us sing there is a green hill far away". Immediately, Joe countered with, "Yes, and you should be on it". I chipped in with a couple of the Cap'n's sayings:-

"Man know thy self. For a woman is forced to"

"There are as many different types of fish in the sea as there are women. And if all the seas were one and made of black ink thy would not be able to write a woman's deception"

The evening gathering ended with tears of laughter instead those of pain and surely one should celebrate a persons' life as much as regret the passing of that person.

My love for Sadie blossomed during these weeks and, just before the festive season, the first of my wedding bans were read. The church I used was the same one where the Cap'n was eulogised so lovingly. At the start of 1988 I spent many hours revising the wedding list and plans. My choice of best man was Gank as he had been there from the first day that I had met Sadie. Marina's partner in business, John, made me a fabulous wedding suit in charcoal grey. Although the bans were read in St. Thomas's my wedding took place in All Saints Church in the centre of Rotherham. Nothing but the best for J. Sadie arrived at the church looking absolutely stunning. She was wearing a full length wedding gown in an ivory and cream coloured material. Gank gave me a wonderful best man's speech at the wedding reception. During the reception an old friend of mine from Meadowbank by the name of Eddie said that a lion had been tamed.

I was very much loved at the time and extremely happy with my lot. My hard work and extensive overtime enabled us to move out of debt and create financial stability. The aim was to set up our love nest ready for the arrival of our firstborn. On the third of June Sadie gave birth to my Son Jason. I was at the sharp end, so as to speak, during the birth and I had the great pleasure of seeing the arrival of Jason. This was the proudest moment of my life. He weighed seven pounds and eight ounce and watching the sight of all the adoring relatives crowded around the hospital cot gave one a sense of deja vu. It was not long before the family Tune arrived back at the love nest to begin the life long journey of family hood.

Who could have imagined that I would be arising during the early hours of the morning to administer a much needed bottle and to change a soaking nappy. I realised early doors that the best way to put a dollop of nappy cream on the correct areas was to take the lid off the bottle and fit his pride and joy in there and twist the jar.

Having an accident at work quickly shattered my euphoria. This meant that the only available income was statuary sick pay, which was a third of my usual earnings. I had arranged to go on holiday with Gank and his new wife Julie. Interestingly enough, they not only became man and wife on my birthday but they named their Son Jay after me. In order to earn a few notes I went round with Daz who was my sister Cheryl's partner. He had a pick up truck and we went round doing the scrap iron bit. As soon as I had enough money off I went on holiday. We went to Cornwall and stayed in a rented chalet. This was a belated honeymoon for both couples and what a time we had. I look back on that holiday with great fondness and I still thank Gank and Julie for the joy of their company.

My feeling of contented euphoria was at an all time high and the run in to Christmas was made even more enjoyable by the fact that this would be baby Jason's first festive season. I returned to my job after my accident only to be laid off due to a lack of work. Even so, the company were still employing casual workers who had not been there as long as me. That was the spur for me to approach my union official to make a claim against the company for negligence. At one time, I would have regarded this as nothing less than spilling the beans but they were picking the fight against me and they were not prepared to do the honourable thing. Once again, the J mentality propelled me to obtain what was rightly mine without resorting to the accepted method. The claim was lodged but on the understanding that this was no quick fix and that I was in for the long haul. So be it. "Bring it on", was my only response to the union official. Principle seems to be a lost attribute nowadays but it has always been my bedrock.

The thoughts of not celebrating Christmas as I would want was the reason for accepting three weeks work in Devon finishing off a demolition job on an old power station. This was the first time that I had worked away since becoming a married man. I missed my family more than I was ever prepared to admit at the time. The money came in very handy and took us into the New Year in some style.

I spent New Years Eve at my Father's house with his second wife Anne and my half sisters. They have always made me feel welcome and still greet me with the unique affection that the family has.

People tend to wish each other all the best and to have a prosperous New Year. Wishing is one thing but there is a thing called reality. The reality of it all was that I was out of work again and scratching around for work. Whilst doing a bit of shopping at a local supermarket I bumped into the Father of my trusted friend Doug from school. His Father was an important member of the union for construction workers. He asked me what I was up to and when I told him I was working as a burner he told me in no uncertain terms that with my intelligence I should be doing a skilled job and not an unskilled job. Acting on his advice I toddled off to the main union office and joined the union on his recommendation. I filled an application form in for a job as a first year improver Steel Erector. This would be the start of my apprenticeship.

The only place where major construction work was happening at the time was in London. I packed my bags, picked up my boots, kissed my family goodbye for now and headed off to the Big Smoke. With complete confidence I went from site to site asking for work. It was just my luck to arrive in London at a time when the construction workers' union had called a major strike. However, a non-union firm from South Wales were finishing a major construction job off on the Isle of Dogs in East London and a foreman for the firm told me that they had a contract coming up at Folkestone in Kent for the Channel Tunnel. I left him my details and low and behold a few days later back in Rotherham I received a phone call asking me to start work on the approach bridges to the Channel Tunnel. Once again, my boots were packed and kisses dispelled. This time, I hooked a small caravan to the back of my car and headed South full of optimism. Hours later, I pulled up at the Blue Cliff caravan park that was teeming with what was known as the tunnel rats. Not the furry variety but with some of the workers it was hard to tell. These guys were the hardest bunch of gruesome blokes that I have encountered. One Irish fellah, who had muscle on muscle and was quite one of the most awesome men that I have ever seen became my close friend during this period of time. He had a heart of gold however and was he was generous to an embarrassing degree. I never confused the issue of niceness with softness. It does not always follow that the nice guys can't do the business.

Paddy, as he was naturally referred to, was to be my main work associate during my stay at Folkestone and taught me many of the ropes in the construction game.

The job lasted six months and I was earning treble what I used to earn at home. There are of course drawbacks and the main one was the lack of home visits. It is all very well earning top money but there is also a thing called family life. I only came home once a month for a long weekend and boy was I tired. I was working twelve hours per day seven days per week.

At Easter, I came home for a few days to have my Son christened in the All Saints Church, Rotherham. I was really proud when the Vicar said that I was flying the flag for Rotherham in his talk to the family gathered around the font. It was a lovely day and the warm feeling of belonging flooded through me once again. We went back to the in-laws for a bite to eat and a few drinks to wet the baby's head. This was a welcome weekend in many respects. All too soon I was packing my boots and air kissing everyone in view. A few hugs later I was driving down the motorway with a lump in my throat. I wanted to make a good start for us and to provide a comfortable basis for our great adventure.

Back at work I found myself working under a general foreman called Patrick. He was yet again another Irishman at the Tranche Manche Link who had come over chasing the money. He sacked more workers than were lost at Flanders. One day, there were ten men guiding a bridge section into place. It was very windy and we were pulling on the ropes like men possessed. Patrick ambled onto the site and with the broadest Irish brogue that I have ever heard said, "Pull you fuckers, you're not taking the dog for a walk". He was full of put downs and sarcasm. One of his favourites was if he caught anybody talking he would say that he was organising a coffee morning with the ladies of Folkestone. I only mention this to show how tough the work was and I stood out like a sore thumb. Many of the workers were very experienced guys and I was the youngest man on the job at the age of twenty-three. The next youngest bloke was aged about forty and it spoke volumes of how hard I was working that Patrick kept me on. His bark was worst than his bite.

To my delight a Rotherham bloke turned up one day by the nickname of Beano. He was so called, because he used to read the Beano comic down the pit before he became an erector. It was good to listen to someone speaking proper English. I used to let him stay in the caravan and share resources. This was called grubbing together and it saved money. I felt that we were a pair of industrial Gypsies. The only fall out we had during this period was his addiction to drink. When he had had a few the inside of the caravan would smell like a rotting corpse on a hot day. I swear that a rat had crawled up his arse and died.

He had a reputation as a bit of a shirker and before long John the gaffer had sussed him out. Beano knew his days were numbered and he decided to go before he was pushed. Beano, being a Rotherham lad, left with some dignity when he went up to John and said, "It's Roy Orbison time". "You what", said John. "It's over", came the reply.

In between times, Sadie had approached the Council for a house for us as we were still in a one bedroom flat. At the time, Gank and Julie had split up and their council house became available. He offered us the chance to have his council house in exchange for our flat. What a bloke. No wonder I still refer to him as my best man. The house was in East Dene and I felt in some ways that I was returning home as I knew a lot of people in the area. Sadie arranged the move and through her efforts the house was fully carpeted and furnished by the time that I had finished the contract and returned to Rotherham. The work on the Channel Tunnel had taken its toll on me and I chilled out for a few weeks getting in plenty of sunbathing in the garden.

During the summer we had the opportunity to have a holiday. Sadie's Mum and Dad took us to the New Forest in Hampshire for a one week's stay. We lodged at one of Sadie's Granddad's connections. The highlight of the week was a trip to the Isle of White. I picked Jason up and showed him the boats coming in. I felt that my boat had truly come in too.

Although I had earned good money funds were beginning to dry up. I decided to sign on at the dole office and duly went down with baby Jason and his Mother on the allotted day. Inside the office I was asked to fill this form in and that form in. Baby Jason was amusing himself by throwing forms all over the place. Suddenly, I thought to myself what the hell am I doing here. With that, I marched the family out of there and swore there and then that I would never sign on the dole again. Later, I went for a drink with my Cousin Tex and discussed the possibility of him arranging work for me as he was a charge hand working at the Rudgely Power Station, in Staffordshire. This meant staying in digs at Stafford whilst I was working on the Power Station. My job was a rigger helping Tex and his team to repair and change valves on the main boilers. I was there from early July until September when I contacted a firm in Basildon, Essex about a possible position as a Steel Erector working in central London. They offered me a job on a construction site at Farringdon Street Station. I accepted the offer and once again my boots were packed and kisses given. The job was the construction of a high rise office block overlooking the station.

I stayed in the Seaman's mission at Poplar in the East End and started the job with a good set of blokes under the guidance of Graham the general foreman. After a couple of weeks I went back to

Rotherham for the weekend. Late on Friday night I eventually arrived back at my house to be greeted by a solemn looking Sadie. She had baby Jason in her arms and she lay down on the bed uttering the famous words that all men should dread. "We need to talk", was her opening comment. No words ever carry such finality as those few words. "I don't love you any more", she said. "Why, is there someone else?" I asked. She assured me that there was no one else and asked me to leave the house straight away and go to my sister's house. With a heavy heart I left and a short while later I was pouring my heart out to my sister Marina. She let me stay in a spare room and told me that I could use it for as long as I needed. I spent hours on the phone to Sadie asking her to reconsider the position but I was isolated in London and I was not having face to face talks. Over the next weeks she became more distant and spent less time talking to me. At the back of mind I was sure that there was someone else involved but she kept up the story that she had simply fell out of love for me. I was still seeing baby Jason at every opportunity and I was still providing Sadie with money for the now splintered family. My work became even more important to me as this was a relief from the torment that I was suffering inwardly. Hairy arsed erectors are not known for their sympathies and I was subjected to bouts of dark humour. One said to me this job creates divorce or piles. Getting a divorce from working away from home and not attending to the wife and, also, suffering piles through sitting on steel girders. Others would repeatedly ask me if the milkman had stopped delivering his rounds.

For the next few months my routine was very predictable. Work all work and return to Rotherham for a few glimpses of baby Jason. My good friend Doug spent a lot of time with me when I returned home and his support meant every thing to me. We patronised a night club called Patches in Rotherham. Doug tried hard to make me see that life must go on and not wallow in self pity or despair. I did not fully understand what he was driving at first but bit by bit his kind words and sound counselling began to sink in. Due to the fact that he is a trusted friend he could say the truth without causing offence. His sympathies and advice given during these dark hours brought much needed stability to my life.

I was still finding it difficult to comprehend though. The house was in first class condition, a baby Son, a well paid job and my love. As far as I was concerned my marriage had not had the chance to blossom and I could not rationalise where Sadie was coming from. Her perceptions of the difficulties in our marriage were not in tandem with mine.

Christmas was approaching and I was filled with new optimism that a few days spent with Sadie would sort out our troubles. This is a time of goodwill to all men but as events turned out I was the only man not to have any goodwill. Sadie was adamant that our marriage had hit the buffers.

Marina kindly fetched baby Jason over to her house where I was staying and I cherished those hours that can never be again. When I returned with baby Jason I asked Sadie once again if there was somebody else. She told me that we had grown apart and that she was entirely on her own.
I asked her to reconsider the position but she said no to any of my suggestions and I was left with no option but to return to Marina's house.

To cheer me up Doug had arranged for us to go to the Patches night club on News Year Eve followed by a party at his brother's girlfriend's house. We eventually ended up at the party to let the New Year in after a pleasant night at the Patches. I went outside for a breath of fresh air when I had the sudden thought to go to Sadie's place. There was a taxi at the bottom of the steps leading to the party and I hopped in and off I went. I arrived at Sadie's house and asked the taxi driver to wait for me. Sadie answered the door but kept the security chain on. "Why can't I come in then"? I asked her. She told me to call back the following day. I thought that this was a little strange as there had not been any animosity between us. Still, I turned round and climbed back into the taxi. For some strange reason the taxi driver set off in the wrong direction. He realised his mistake and proceeded to turn round in the middle of the road. That provided me with the chance to espy a van parked in a side street. The van had a padlock on the back doors. The only van that I knew of that looked like this belonged to none other than Gasping Gaz.

That was it. I screamed to the taxi driver to stop and I threw a hand full of notes in his direction. After rapping my knuckles on the door of my house I shouted to Sadie to send the snake out. There was a muffled silence inside followed by sounds of people scampering about. The door opened with my magic key and I entered like a gunfighter on a mission into a Wild West saloon. Gasping Gaz dashed down the stairs and attempted a Kung Fu style kick to my chest. He bounced off me and landed on his back. Being a gentleman I picked him up and then re christened him at that moment on from Gary to Gasping Gaz. The song, 'All I want for Christmas is my two front teeth', flashed through my mind. Sadie tried telling me that he had turned up the worst for wear and that he was staying in the back bedroom. My derision knew no bounds. He will be staying in hospital more like was my retort. The sounds of baby Jason whimpering in his sleep was enough for me to leave the house and the sorrow mess that it had become.

Gasping Gaz at a later stage admitted adultery and I divorced Sadie on those grounds.

Chapter 22: Single, Free and Available

In early January, 1990 I went to a Rotherham solicitor and petitioned for a divorce. The divorced became a costly event in terms of money but more importantly the loss of access to baby Jason. In terms of the money it was well spent and I regarded it as the removal of two bad apples from my life. An ex-friend and an ex-wife. Any one who has been through a divorce will tell their story and it will always be slightly different to some one else's. I began to look for positives in my life and listed them. At the top of my list was baby Jason. If nothing being the Father of Jason was the greatest thing that I have achieved. It soon became obvious to me that she was not the queen for this king. Some people take years to overcome their divorce but life is for living not dwelling.

I returned to London with a heavy heart but with a feeling of some relief. The contract at Farringdon Street was coming to an end and quite a few of the workers were being paid off. I was called into the office and I was told that I was a good improver erector and I was offered a contract on the Canary Wharf project. One night I was in a pub down Bow way and I struck up a conversation with an old man called Johnny Greenhall. He was a rough old stick but he had plenty of chat. He asked me what I did and I told him that I was staying at the Seaman's Mission. When I said that I was thinking of moving out he suggested that I rented a spare room from him. He was on his own with only a dog for company. This seemed to be a good arrangement for both of us. He earned a few notes and I was sleeping in comfortable lodgings at Stepney just off Commercial Road. Johnny was a great bloke and he loved his tot of rum. He told me one night that there were plenty of fish in the sea and that I aught to go out and enjoy myself.

I stayed down London one weekend and I went to Petty coat Lane market and bought myself some nice clothes. After a shave and shampoo I was looking something like. That night I went to Kitsons at Bow. This was a famous dance hall and renowned for being a meeting place for singles and divorced people. I wandered around the dance hall looking at the available talent and began to feel very pleased with myself. During the evening I propped myself up at the bar enjoying a rare beer when a girl approached me and said that her friend would like to have a drink with me. "O.K.", said I. "Where is she"? That was that. Lorraine and I became more than just good friends and we were together for a couple of months. To my enjoyment she was an Elvis Presley fan and she had a pair of knockers that would grace any top shelf magazine. She was a lovely girl with typical Irish warmth. My time spent with her was extremely enjoyable and I have nothing but fond memories of her. She went to Ireland on an extended holiday and I met someone else at work. Her name was Mandy and she worked in the works canteen. After three or four days she sussed me out that I was giving her bull shit. She said to me, "If you are a constructional engineer J then why are you smoking my cigarettes, drinking my drinks and had been living in the Seaman's Mission"? I had been caught out and decided to move on.

My old mate Beano reared his ugly head again and before long we were strutting our stuff down the Elephant and Castle. We spent our time having a few beers, talking about old times and trying to pull any bird who did not ask us 'what the time is' first. The night we decided to go the Seven Sisters pub at Aldgate marked a decline in our friendship. He had been bragging about a red head who worked behind the bar. He told me that he was chatting her up and that she was there for the taking. So, we went down to the pub to check her out. "Hello Darling", said I. "My name is J and I am yours". With that, she grinned broadly and nodded when I suggested that we met up for a drink sometime. Beano went ballistic. His favourite motto was every man for himself. Not so when it was turned on him. His parting comment was along the lines of, "You dirty twat. She was mine". "Yes", I thought. "In your dreams". Claire and I met up a couple of nights later and we had a pleasant drink and a bite to eat. We went back to her place for the afters. I was knocking her off until the end of May.

The divorce was beginning to take its toll and I was spending more and more time sorting out the legalities. Claire, quite understandably, was demanding more of my time and I was not keeping the commitment. It was not a surprise, therefore, that she told me it was over. Apparently, she did not trust me when I went home and she was not entirely convinced that it was all over between my wife and me. Of course, it was. Not with the other ladies though.

One door closes and another bedroom door opens.

I decided to have a week off work in order to finalise the divorce proceedings and tie up the legal requirements. Big Bob came round and in his usual stage whisper bellowed that we should go out and that he would show me a good time. I blinked in amazement at his terminology but accepted the gesture as that of a true friend. He was on something of a roll as he had bedded a few women, some who still had a pulse, and he had become a Don Juan of Rotherham. Although the nights were good the daytime spent seeing solicitors and the rest of the people who have their hand stretched out was not going so well.

This week off work has stuck in my mind as the Blanket week. One night, Big Bob and I picked up two likely girls and eventually we were invited to spend the night at the house of the girl I was with. How it happened I cannot recall but the next thing that I knew was Big Bob shouting up the stair well for a blanket. Apparently, his girl had taken off and he wanted to crash out on the settee. I threw him a blanket down and I went back to clean sheets, duvet cover and company. The problem was that this was the third time that it happened that week. Hey brother can you spare me a blanket. I began to think that Big Bob was a Red Indian sitting it out on a reservation somewhere.

All too soon it was back to work and the joy of sitting on a girder a few hundred feet up in the air.

Marina, meanwhile, had been negotiating for access for me with little Jason. For a while it was working quite well and I came home every weekend to see him. His second birthday came and went but there was always an undercurrent to this arrangement and it was not long before the deep resentments rose like a monster in Loch Ness. I had been picking little Jason up from his Grandparent's and they were tired of being the piggy's in the middle. Access was becoming more difficult so I went to my solicitor to have a legally binding arrangement. Unfortunately, little did I know that I had inadvertently started one of Rotherham's longest custody battles. Every single aspect of my past and present life was suddenly placed under the legal microscope. It has taken too long for the rights of Fathers to be taken into consideration and judging by the campaigning of Fathers for Justice I am not sure that as a society that we have progressed much. Before I knew it I was on the train back to the Big Smoke and it would be fourteen long years before I saw my beloved Son again.

I was determined never to give up the belief that I would know my Son again and his presence was a burning ache in my chest.

My work became my escape and I gave my all every day. The Company were magnificent with their support and I cannot speak too highly of their staff/management technique. Around August time I came down to Rotherham for a long weekend on the say so of the site manager. Naturally, I sought out my friends as soon as my bag had been dropped off at Marina's. Big Bob, Doug and I found ourselves at a notorious pick up place on the outskirts of Rotherham. Doug had shot up and he was now clearing the ground at a height of six feet and four inches. He was eighteen stone of solid muscle not counting the gristle. Big Bob and I were now six feet tall and looking like two bank safes and just as hard. What a trio. All night long we were surrounded by an assortment of dolls and some were more than just interested. Big Bob sidled up to me and said, "What's up with you. She is wetter than a fishmongers slab". I just shrugged my shoulders and Big Bob just never saw what I saw. The bouncers were positioning themselves around us and I had the feeling that all was not well. There were nine or ten of them and it went through my mind that I did not know why they were targeting us. Out of the corner of my eye I saw a girl that I had previously rejected literally crawling over one of the bouncers like an outbreak of measles. I put a cigarette in my mouth and went up to the bouncer in question. He offered me a light with a cigarette lighter and at that point the music stopped. I reared back and head butted him like a mad bull gorging a hated matador. His lights went out in a spectacular manner. That was it. Big Bob was rolling on the floor with one of the bouncers. Doug had another one up against a wall. I was not sure if he was hitting him or plastering the wall with him. They waded into us with chairs and then I realised this one was for keeps. My old friend adrenaline flowed and the vein on my neck stuck out like a drainpipe. Chairs, tables, fists, feet just about everything went that night. My last clear thought was tickling the goolies of one of them with the toe end of my brogues. Days later some one asked me how I knew what order I ran the fight in and was I aware which one to hit next. Silly question really. The biggest goes first and then it is descending order. A fight in a Wild West saloon could never have matched the ferocity of that night. There is a famous film called 'Last Man Standing' only in this case it was the Last Three standing, us.

We piled out but not before we collected our coats from the checkout lady. Big Bob picked up his coat, turned round and said, "Any one for marbles"?

Our mob burst through the doors and vacated the scene at a fast rate. To our relief, there was a taxi waiting. We climbed into the back of the taxi and gave the necessary directions. When our taxi turned the first corner, with us looking over our shoulders through the rear windscreen, the first of the boys in blue 'nick nick' cars screamed round the corner heading towards the club. The taxi stopped at Big Bob's flat, in Eastwood. We went into his flat laughing our heads off. In the bathroom we examined the damage to ourselves. Doug had a right shiner and a three inch gash down his forehead. Big Bob had the other marble player's teeth marks on his face. Typical of Big Bob though; the pain had not started. I had cuts, bruises and more bumps than a busy road full of traffic calmers. More to my annoyance I noticed that my belcher gold chain was missing. Of course, I went into a rant and swore that I would never lose a chain again in a fight. Doug, meanwhile, was in the kitchen making a pot of tea. At this moment the doorbell rang. Big Bob opened the door and in came one of Big Bob's girls. These women of his were always referred to as a half past two bird. Well, lets face it, what sort of woman is still in a club at half fast two. The cleaner would probably be worth more of one.

She breezed in and told us that we were big boys and "OOOOOH, aren't you built big". At that, we stripped off to the waist and began to pose as if we were at a body builder's convention. The girl went into the bedroom and lay down on the bed. She whipped her kit off and began a D.I.Y sex session. Doug took one look at the way she was doing this and afterwards called her the Banjo Player. Normally, this would be a turn on but who in their right mind would follow Big Bob.

Back in London the job was coming to an end and the rumour control board was in full swing. The company I was working for had been taken over and it was rumoured that some of us were facing redundancy. Not one for being too depressed by such tittle-tattle I went down to Kitson's dancehall at Bow for a look round and a sniff of the air. I suppose you have guessed by now. She was size 12, petite and as blonde as they come. And come she did. Babs was a nurse in a private hospital and I can assure you there was nothing wrong with her bedside techniques. On the first time I met her she put her foot on my shoulder and smiled at me. "Whoa", I said. "How about both of them". She grinned even more. We were together right up to the end of November when the bad news about the company hit us hard. I had no option but to kiss her goodbye and leave for Rotherham. On reflection just how good is the 'if only bit'. I should have stayed with her and tried my luck in London. By the time I was passing Leicester the regrets were diminishing and thoughts of Rotherham began to fill my head again. Within days of being back Doug's Dad phoned me up and referred me to a construction firm from Cleveland. I spoke to them and they offered me a job on a construction site at one of Sheffield's largest stainless steel producers. This was just before Christmas and the goodwill feeling that miracles, albeit minor, can give you swept over me.

Chapter 23: Relapse (or to hell with drugs)

This feeling of euphoria eventually proved to be costly. I teamed up with a couple of old associates and before long I took some amphetamines. Even now I cannot justify why I did it. I offer no excuses only to say that it was completely foolish of me to descend into the chemical world of drugs. For a short while the pain of my marital troubles were eased until the turn of the New Year. On the morning of the third of January, 1991 I was in what was known as the basket (a safety device when high off the ground) bolting some girders together. I looked down and I saw Big Bob and a mate of his nicknamed Ziggy walking towards me. Big Bob had an expression on his face like I have never seen. A quick signal to the hoist man and I was down on the ground shaking Big Bob and yelling at him to tell me what had happened. He told me that my brother David had hung himself. I sank to my knees clutching my head. My mouth was wide opened but the screams were in my head. Never have I felt so alone and so completely ill with grief. The works foreman knew what had happened and he told me to take a fortnight off work. I asked Ziggy to take a note to my Dad's house and I went straight round to my Mum's house. The family told me that David had hung himself at Samantha's house. He had stood on a trestle at the top of the stairs and launched himself into the only escape that he knew. I began to berate myself that I had not helped him enough when he was feeling low. Just how low he was is any one's guess. I still ponder on what it was that tipped his balance of rational decision making to make him take that step.

My self esteem was so low that I turned to the chemical solution. Totally wrong. There are many ways of dealing with situations that peg you back but to take drugs is not the answer. For every high that the drugs give you there are ten lows as well.

The day of the funeral was the usual January dismal day. We all turned up in our finery to see David off. St. Thomas's church was full of well wishers and people offering their respect. My recollections of the service are patchy but I do remember that we sang 'The Lord is my Shepherd' and it was then that the lumps in the throat were evident. The loss of the Cap'n was something but this was beyond me. David was only twenty-four when he passed away but he has never left me.

I am convinced that if David could pass me a message he would tell me to be strong not only for my sake but for the sake of the family.

The wake was held in East Herringthorpe Workingman's Club in Rotherham. Quite a few of my extended family are members of this club and I am still a member of the sports division within the club. Speeches were said and hugs and handshakes seemed to be the order of the day. Of course, there were a few pints being lowered or raised in memory of David and the atmosphere slowly but inevitably changed as the afternoon wore on. The mumblings of how are you and tributes to David were replaced by doubt and questions. In corners the sounds of impromptu inquests filled the air. My mood became more sullen underpinned with a deep anger and the frustration of not knowing why. Recurring feelings of not being there for him washed over me but as the saying goes you 'cannot put old head on young shoulders'. As is the way of these things in darkest Rotherham, the conversation turned once again but to matters of male machoism and scapegoats. Someone mentioned that David was alright before he began to associate with a mob from Blackburn on the other side of Rotherham. Other people muttered that this mob was handling more pot than an army kitchen. In one of those times when suddenly there is a pause in proceedings a voice was heard to say that Gasping Gaz had been seen at the funeral. Gasping was from Blackburn and at the mention of his name and Blackburn in the same conversation was enough for me to bellow out, "Taxi, now". Naturally, the weak hearted mourners started to persuade me not to do anything rash but Big Bob and my friend Doug took no heed and we set off to a pub in the Blackburn area when the taxi arrived. The pub was known by the locals as the Swamp. Judging by the low life that resided in there it was aptly named. Within twenty minutes the taxi pulled up outside the Swamp and we stood in a line like desperados who had come to town for a showdown.

Big Bob had been a work mate of Gasping Gaz but on the way to the Swamp he told me that his allegiance was with me and f*** the Gasping t*** and his cronies. Big Bob and Doug went into the Swamp and I stood outside on dry land. Doug twisted his neck like Mike Tyson and pushed the door open with an imaginary hand on his holster. For what seemed an eternity all was quiet. I learnt later during the match analysis that Doug had managed to have everybody quiet and seated. Big Bob was talking to a few of them. As far as Big Bob and Doug were concerned it was enough that they had shown their faces in such a dump. Of course, I did not know what was happening so I wiped my feet and entered the pub. At that precise moment Big Bob was accusing Gasping Gaz that he was a grass and a back stabber. He asked Gasping Gaz to repeat what he had been putting about. At the sound of the door creaking open all eyes turned to me. All doubt was removed from the assembled brain cells in the heads of the Swamp inhabitants. They knew that a visit had become business, meaningful business.

Doug spun round to look at me and was promptly hit on his back with a pool cue held by a non-entity called Millie. He was sent to his particular escape point by Doug. One tremendous punch sent Millie over the pool table. Not a ball was disturbed. Poor shot thought I. He should have pocketed the number 6 ball. Doug turned round to glare at the flock and quietly said, "Rack them up again". Showtime. I immediately picked Gasping Gaz and his brother up. His brother was known as the Milky Bar Kid. So named because he was white skinned, wore glasses and about as useful. It was rumoured that they used to sleep in the same bed together when they were kids so I introduced them to each other once again. I banged their heads together with as much power that I could muster. Gasping Gaz's false teeth shot out like a snakes tongue having a tasty snack His brother momentarily stood like a wilted flower with his head hanging down. They both hit the floor in a heap. After that it was just pure mayhem. The noise of fists hitting jaws sounded as if someone had set off indoor fireworks. Big Bob was doing the sweeping up. Anyone still standing or had been missed by me and Doug was cleared out of the room by Big Bob. At the end of the showdown Doug turned round to me and said, "Some f******* games room". To my surprise Doug went up to the landlord and offered to pay. "What the hell are you doing", I asked him. Doug told the landlord that there would be enough in the pockets of the fallen unclassified.

We went outside and Big Bob suggested that we went for a celebratory drink in another local pub. The lights had been switched off and the door locked to make us think that they were shut in case we went in. Doug knocked on the door and I assured them that we would cause no trouble. If nothing else, my word was always known as my bond. The door was unlocked and in we went.

Big Bob, being Big Bob, had not read the script. My word was not his word. As soon as he adjusted his eyes to the gloom he spotted a guy called Nick. Apparently, this guy owed Big Bob some money and he had also done Big Bob out of some highly paid work. Big Bob was in no mood to take prisoners. One hit and down went Nick. Doug and I immediately ushered Big Bob out of the pub.

So, in the aftermath of all this when we were reliving the fight and who did what to who Big Bob grinned and said, "Yeah. We were that good that we couldn't even get a drink".

Chapter 24: Quiet Times (by my standards)

The job at the stainless steel factory was going well but the blot on the landscape was my housing situation. I was living, no, existing in a bed sit in the Broom Valley area of town. In the middle of February I received notification the long awaited operation on my leg was to take place. This was due to the industrial accident that I had had on the demolition a few years previous. My stay in hospital lasted a week and thankfully the operation proved to be very successful. On my discharge I went to my Mother's house for a small period of convalescence. She suggested to me that I left my bed sit and moved back with her. Even so, I had put my name down with the council for my own two bed-roomed flat. I was still hoping to have some where of my own so that my Son Jason could stay with me. My Mother was rarely in. She had taken the loss of David really badly as we all did. It is every parent's worst nightmare to outlive a child of theirs.

Whilst I was off work my friend Doug's Dad had a whip round for me at work and to my complete surprise. This was a lovely gesture and one that I have never forgotten since. My love life was going well too. Her name was Sandra and for a change she was a brunette. This relationship lasted until Christmas of that year. She had a lot to put up with though. I was still struggling with the loss of Dave and the loss of my Son. Sandra listened to my woes and gave me as much support as she could.

During this lull in my life I was dealt a body blow with the news that my nephew Luke's Uncle had been stabbed to death at a party in Sheffield. The Uncle's name was Tony and he had been a good friend of the family. He was a sad loss to everyone who knew him well.

On Remembrance Day I was offered my current flat. I was really pleased with the flat and it suited my every needs; apart from not seeing Jason that is. Bit by bit I added to the furnishings in the flat and it soon became home. My Mother was sad to see me go as she had come to rely on my support and help. Bless her, she popped round to my flat when she could and she often did a bit of cleaning and tidying up.

At Christmas of 1991 Sandra and I parted company. We are on friendly terms even now but the amount of whizz that I was taking was too much for her. The mood swings and excuses had increased to such a level that she did not want my life style any more. I could not offer her what she wanted from the relationship.

Christmas came and went and I started out the New Year arm in arm with a girl called Melanie. She came from the Blackburn estate, scene of the draining of the Swamp, very near to where Gasping Gaz had set up home with my ex-wife Sadie and my Son Jason. It was heart breaking sometimes going down to Blackburn knowing that I was so close to Jason but a million miles away. I used to ask people who knew us both how Jason was going on and of his well being. The only consolation that I could gain from this situation was the memory of Gasping Gaz's teeth heading south. Unfortunately, although Melanie was a fine girl, the misery of going down to her estate proved too much for me and we soon said our goodbyes.

Continuing the desire not to settle for the usual petite, blonde and bluey green eyes I met up with a red head from my not too distant past. Buxom was hardly in it where she was concerned. If she did a back flip she would end up with black eyes. It is always good to have a lady on one's arm on Valentine's Day. "Do you love me"? she asked. "I give you one don't I", I replied. And thus was the state of our relationship set in stone. She worked at a local nut factory and I presumed she gained the job on her own status. Our love affair misfired until the summer months until I caught her in what looked like an arrangement with a known drug addict. It was probably in all innocence but I was completely mistrustful of anyone from that crowd. Just because I was still dabbling in the odd intake it did not mean to say that I was prepared to tolerate any-one else's habits. How ever hypocritical that may sound in the end I have my standards. Later, I found out that she had been seeing a guy called Dennis and not as a member of the knitting club. As the saying goes, it takes two to tango.

Funny how these things turn out though. She looks really well nowadays and I would not kick her out of bed on a winter's day. Not until she has paid back the money she owes me.

I was just about holding a job down but my speed consumption was beginning to increase. Dependency levels rise, as the buzz from a smaller dose is not giving the same effect. Due to the turmoil that my life was in I became more and more dysfunctional. Bills were not paid in order to fund my plunge into mock escapism. It came as no surprise that I ended up back in hospital.

I had gone to the hospital to visit a friend who was recovering from acute anxiety attacks. Whilst I was meandering down the corridor leading away from his ward I literally bumped into Dr. Prescott. She took one look at me and her alarm bells rang. Apparently, she asked me if I was all right and my response was to mumble incoherently at her. She told me at a later stage that I bounced down the corridor like an out of control pinball. Later, a loud hammering on my door waked me up. Waiting for me was a paramedic vehicle with a social worker. They quietly advised me to grab a few things and go with them for some rest. I knew the game was up and that I had exhausted my ability to cope.

On my arrival at hospital a line of Psychiatric Nurses were there to greet me. The welcome committee was positioned in staggered arrangement in case I kicked off or ran off. They need not have bothered themselves, as I was too weak to act.

I sauntered down the ward looking for familiar faces and where to lay my head. Unbeknown to me, the hospital had some sort of partnership with the Doncaster Health Authority and because Rotherham Hospital was full I was to be transferred to Doncaster. Before long, I was in a hospital taxi surrounded by four heavies who had come along for the ride just in case I objected to the grand day out. I wondered where the hell they were taking me but a voice in the taxi kept reassuring me that I was going somewhere nice and that I would be fine. As it was they were right. My stay in Doncaster was brilliant and I have nothing but praise for all the staff who worked there. The delivery of the treatment of patients had come a long way since my first encounter with the medical system. For the first time I felt that the hospital staff were heaven bent on placing as much trust as they could in me and I responded positively to their ethos.

The hospital had a self selection menu at meal times. In addition, patients were allowed to wear their own clothing during the day. After a period of time the staff would give selected patients enough money to enable them to go to their home for a day visit.

On one occasion, I was given a lift back to Doncaster by a so called female friend. Unfortunately, her car broke down near Doncaster railway station. She asked me for help but I was forced into admitting that I was a patient at Doncaster Hospital and that I had to return there by ten O'clock for medication. Her partner was a friend of Gasping Gaz and it did not take too long before the news of my circumstances was relayed back. This nugget of information was used frequently afterwards whenever my ex-wife wanted verbal ammunition to spit at me. Within what seemed no time at all I had made a recovery and the parting words of one of the nurses was that I had arrived with four heavies in tow and that I had been a gentle pussycat throughout.

The hospital asked me if I required any after care when I left the hospital but I naively decided to refuse their offer of help. This was to prove a huge mistake and in retrospect I should have taken advantage of their offer. I obtained a job erecting down at Silvertown in London and everyone in my family said that I had gone back to work too soon after my emotional trauma.

This job lasted a couple of months and was memorable for my heroics. One of the lads on the site was an old school friend of mine. Adam and myself were one hundred and eighty feet in the air knocking down girders with a sledgehammer. It was the safety rule that the person using the hammer should be wearing a safety harness that was clipped onto the aerial basket. Adam took over the hammering duties but forgot to clip the safety harness in the correct slot. He swung the hammer and disappeared over the edge with the momentum of the blow. I lunged forward and caught him around his waist and dragged him back. "Thanks for that", he said, "I am on the promise this weekend". This could have been one breakdown to another.

Chapter 25: Suffering in the Smoke

This particular time in London was one hard drag. There was hardly any time for entertainment to alleviate the daily grind of work, bed and more work. At every opportunity I was on a pay phone to enquire about Jason and my sister Marina, bless her, was my go between to ferret out details and news. Unfortunately, it was a case of 'King Canute' where I was concerned. I was banging my head against a brick wall and I was being engulfed like a Tsunami. No news is good news as they say but no news only served to raise my anxieties. Days became weeks became months. By the time the contract was coming to a close it was time to celebrate my birthday. Or so I thought. It was one of the most miserable birthdays that I can remember. I returned to Rotherham full of hope and expectations but these were soon dashed as my ex-wife refused to allow me any contact with Jason. The courts, as is the way of these things, were dragging their heels and no definitive answer was available.

My unrealistic enthusiasm soon turned to depression and the clouds of darkness began to descend. It is, therefore, no shock to recall that waiting for me one night was my old associate 'The Doc'. "Just a bit", I said, "To get me through this night". Of course, I knew and so did he that this night meant next week and the one after. Before long, we were travelling as far as Doncaster in search of the white powder. Once again, I embraced the chemical scene and the false escapes it offered. Work was intermittent and I ended up earning a crust here and a few bob there. This was the pattern of events for the remainder of the year but there were one or two little incidents to liven up the memories.

I had a number of interesting dates but one lady stands out in more ways than one. This lady who was called Peroxide Pat was having a drink in a Rotherham Town centre pub. Naturally, my predator instincts kicked in at the sight of a petite, blonde and buxom woman. The grin was flashed and any lingering doubt removed. With a smile we left the pub and went back to her place up Kimberworth Park. We had no sooner settled down on the settee than she asked me if I wanted a drink of coffee. She bobbed off and returned with a cup. Without saying a word she put a long-playing record on and went up stairs. I sipped my coffee and to my disgust it was clock cold. The record finished and I heard her yell out to me. With complete puzzlement at her erratic behaviour I went to the bottom of the stairs and to my delight she was standing on the top step wearing bugger all but a Mickey Mouse Tee shirt. She looked at me and said, "Your coffee is cold, the record is finished and I am nearly naked. What is your problem?" Up I went.

I had been in the house for less than six minutes and the action had begun. Even by my standards that was going some. The following morning found me semi skipping down the street polishing my nails on my coat with a smug grin on my face.

A few days later I was in my flat and to my astonishment there was a clothes prop being banged against my bedroom window. I went downstairs to the outside door and on the doorstep was a friend of Peroxide Pat called Dot. She explained that Pat had told her that I was horny stuff and that she had come round for some. Up we went but without a Tee shirt.

Nearer to Christmas Big Bob came round to my flat and said to me that it was about time I kicked the Billy (whizz) into touch. He invited me to go with him to a party held by an old friend in one of the districts largest pubs. He was in the scrap metal business and the pub was close by to his place of work. I dutifully turned up at the appointed place well scrubbed and tidy. In the seething mass was a contingent from a rival family scrap firm called the Pritchards. During the evening one of the Pritchards stood up and started having some banter with our host. Big Bob went over to him and told him to pick on some one his own size like Big Bob for instance. The expected outcome to a retort like that was duly delivered and Big Bob shot backwards with the force of the punch that was landed on his face. For once, I decided to let Big Bob have his fun and I went to the toilet to fill the beds of Blackburn. Suddenly, the toilet door burst open and in came three of the aggrieved firm and gave me a good whacking. I struggled to my feet and made for the exit. Big Bob was outside already looking the worst for wear. At that precise moment Big Bob's date for the evening arrived in a taxi. "What the hell is going on", she screamed. I gave her a potted version of the events and she accused us of being two spineless gets. "You are going to let them get away with that?" My pride welled up and in I went. The pub should have been renamed The Slaughterhouse.

By the time I had finished, the bodies were piled one on top of another. If you did not know any better you would have thought that you had stumbled into an abattoir. It had been a bridge too far for Big Bob but not for me. For a long time afterwards when the lads met for a drink and recalled this story the fight was referred as The Heavy Metal Scrap.

The next day we ventured down to the pub and to our surprise there was half a Guinness bottle stuck in the wall. Apparently, when I went back into the arena Big Bob's date followed me and went for someone with the bottle. It was rumoured that she launched one muppet by cracking the bottle over the top of his head. How the bottle ended up in the wall is anybody's guess.

As this firm originated from Sheffield I was told later that word of J. Tune had spread across the border and that I was being talked about as someone to avoid.

It is said that what goes up comes down and so it proved. My lift from such a battle evaporated totally on New Years Eve. Three of us had ventured over to Barnsley in search of something to take and there was absolutely naff all. Someone suggested to us that some guy in Doncaster would be able to help us out. Off we went to the address that we had been given. We spent ages in a cold, freezing asbestos garage waiting for a dealer to turn up. He must have dealt his last hand, as he did not show. Cutting our losses we set off back to Rotherham. Two girls were walking along and thumbed a lift. Our luck is in here I thought but that was soon dashed as they legged it as soon as we reached the place they had directed us to. We lost sight of them in the middle of a Doncaster estate that was twinned with Beirut. What a night, I don't think so. We arrived back in Rotherham looking sicker than a Blackpool donkey. Fancy having Cold Turkey on New Year's Eve?

Chapter 26: One Mad Year

1993 was met with bleary eyes and an ache for some whizz. When my senses finally kicked in I realised that I was in a flat in the Burngreave area of Sheffield. How I ended up there when I was supposed to be in Rotherham is anybody's guess. Apparently, I had all but crashed when some bright spark decided to go to Sheffield in one final search for some action. My breakfast consisted of a fix that could have launched a Saturn rocket. Happy New Year was probably the last sensible thought that went through my head. After that it was the chemical cocktail that rushed through. The feeling lasted most of the day and into the night. As is the way of these things, there is always a reaction to the rush. For my grand feeling of euphoria I was to experience many lows. My need for the dependency prevented me from fully exploring the side effects of this assault on back street drugs. The worse thing had to be taking sleeping tablets to come down from a high but I even started to give them a miss.

No matter which way anyone looked at it I was gone. My weight just dropped off through a severe lack of food and the extreme hyper activity that I was suffering.

It is so difficult in these circumstances to define the thin line between sanity and the assumption of being sane.

For most of January I was bang at it, to use the common jargon, but a sad event towards the end of the month slowed me up. The Father of my sister Marina's Son Dominic died suddenly and without any warning. At the age of thirty-three he died of a stroke. He had been ill but no one realised just how unwell he really was. The news hit me hard and I used the excuse to fill up my shopping basket with more chemical goodies. Of course, I was looking for an escape from the tragedies of life, mine especially, and drugs seemed to be the only avenue open to me. More like a cul-de-sac if the truth were known.

Samantha never turned me away from her doorstep and I enjoyed playing football with my nephews Luke and our David's lad Daniel.

Across the road from Samantha lived my Mother but her attitude was one of keeping me at arm's length with a few choice comments thrown in. My relationship with my Mother diminished drastically as she quite rightly had no time for her Son being on drugs.

Doc and I went over to Burngreave, Sheffield one day to score some whizz. The, and I use the term loosely, gentlemen doing the deal stated the price that they wanted. I received the bag of amphetamines and handed over the money. Doc meanwhile was waiting in the car with the engine running. As I was leaving one of the stone faced dealers cried out that I had not paid enough. Another one picked up a shortened baseball bat and came at me. Enough said. The vein in my neck stood out in its customary manner and suddenly it was show time. I rushed at them like a raging bull and decked two of them before they knew what had happened. The other two took a hit and ran. I picked up the money that they had dropped and dashed off to the car. No Doc. Where the hell was he? I looked down the road and he was at the traffic lights waiting for the lights to turn to green. The cowardly little turd. I made up the distance in double quick time and bellowed at him to slide over and I took the wheel. With a roar of the engine and enough smoke to make a drag car racer envious I high tailed for the sanctuary of Rotherham. When I reached Rotherham Doc asked me where I was going. I replied that we were going to the Casualty Unit of the General Hospital. Naturally, he asked why. At that moment I pulled up outside the and turned to him and said, "To put you in there." With that I hit him with one almighty punch and dragged him out of the car. I dumped him in the doorway of the Casualty Unit and calmly departed back to my flat.

A few days later the buxom red head contacted me out of the blue to offer me sex in return for a bit of speed. She told me that her partner was not doing much for her and that he was at his Mother's house cutting her grass. I told her that she had not returned the money that she owed me from a previous loan that I had given her and that I did not paddle in other people's muck. No matter what there are enough women going round without having someone else's cast offs. As I had not forgotten about her performing round the back of a Blues Club in Sheffield one night I felt that justice had been served.

At Easter to celebrate Big Bob's birthday we went to the Zoo pub in Rotherham. He had previously been involved in a fight with a notorious Rotherham family nicknamed the Cream Bun's for some reason or other. Of course, Big Bob being Big Bob had not bothered to tell me this piece of news until we were literally stood outside the pub. "O.K.", said I, "I will watch your back you just do what a man has got to do". Even as I was saying this I thought I sounded like an angry cowboy in a Western movie. With this thought still rattling around my brain we pushed our way through the swing doors and held our fists by our sides like two mean gunslingers.

The elder Cream Bun was sitting on a stool drinking of all things a pint of orange cordial. Big Bob drove at him and threw the deliverance punch. Just as he was doing that, the Cream Bun slid down slightly on the stool that he was sitting on. Big Bob missed by a country mile and fell on the top of him. They began to roll around the floor like two over sexed wart hogs. Grunting and panting with steamy snorts coming thick and fast. Whilst this was going on I was telling the rest of the assembled Muppets to keep their distance and to stay out of it. To my surprise a huge guy came at both of them brandishing a stool over his head. What I did not know was that the landlord of the pub had hired this guy as a bouncer in an effort to have some degree of order in the place. Well, I swung a left hook and caught him as well as old Henry caught Mohammed Ali. Down he went in a heap near the door. Big Bob and the elder Cream Bun had dragged themselves to a standing position and I told them to go outside and finish their business across the road in a quiet area behind the shops. Off they went with me as master of ceremonies. Eventually, they agreed to put the business to bed and shook hands. As it turned out they became good mates and Big Bob even took his sister out for a while and anything he could get. We returned to the pub and the bouncer was sitting on the floor wailing something about him being from Sheffield and what was happening. I growled at him that he would be in hospital if he did not shut up. The landlord met us at the doorway with an Alsatian dog at the end of a very short lead. I told him that things were fine and that they had shook hands and that we were coming back in for a drink. He announced that I was barred. "You what", I screamed. I moved forward and gave him my best Lower Kimberworth kiss. "I am barred now you twat".

One week later, just to show my regard for the ban, I went into the Zoo pub for a quick pint and a gossip. Predictably, the barman refused to serve me so I sent a gofer to the bar for my drink. The landlord spotted me drinking his health and said, "There is no stopping you is there?" Point taken. What the hell was he going to do? Send for the police? Risk a kick-off? I don't think so. That, then, was my one and only ban and it lasted a whole week. As it turned out, years later I gave his ex-wife one.

Now that the ban was lifted I soon settled into a routine of calling into the Zoo for a drink and a chat with the lads. So it was that I was to be found in one corner of the pub talking to a couple of the East Dene Mafia brigade and a couple of notables by way of Tigger and Dec. Just as I was slurping my way through the second pint the door of the pub opened and the guy who came in brushed both door jams at the same time with his shoulders. Six foot something and still disappearing. Ginger hair, from Gypsy stock, giving rise to his name of Ginna Mish. He was a Ginna on a mission to do damage. His gimmick was to go around offering five hundred pounds to anyone who lay him low. He grabbed Tigger and moved him to one side like a fly being swatted with a newspaper. The floorboards shuddered as he came over to my corner and spoke in a low gravely voice. "'Ave me and thee a problem here?". I looked up at him and thought to myself that I have never seen an oak tree move. Obviously, he was unaware that the song 'I'm a lumberjack and I'm alright' entered my head. It was time to fell the oak tree. As he was leaning down to vaporise me with his foul breath I reached up and grabbed him by the lapels. Whoosh. Straight onto my head. Without missing a beat I introduced my knee to his nose and off we went. The next few moments are still a blur in my memory but what I do know is that the fight we had, which I thought was in one corner only, had spread all over the pub. I became aware that the entire clientele of the pub were standing on the benches that ran around the walls. Broken tables, smashed glasses and general mayhem seemed to be the order of the day. Ginna Mish was just a sprawled mass on the floor. In truth, he looked like a bull walrus having a sun bathe.

Of course, the boys in blue appeared as I was picking shards of glass out of my arms. "Who has been fighting here then", one of them asked. 'Not me', came the universal reply. Just like a scene from Spartacus. Meanwhile, I escaped through the fire exit whistling the tune from 'The Great Escape' film.

This fight was known as the fight of the century throughout the boroughs of Rotherham. My stock was at an all time high. The next time my voice was heard in the Zoo it was to pronounce that the drinks were on me.

My love life was ticking over quite nicely. I was with a girl called Avril who worked in a chemist's shop. At least my condoms were to be had for free. I don't suppose the shop did not do too well during that time. Lovely girl was Avril but as soon as she became aware of my reputation she started to cool off romantically. Should you ever read this account Avril let me tell you that I thought the world of you.

To be honest, I have always assumed that Avril found out that I was handling more drugs than the chemist shop was dispensing.

The drug taking was becoming out of control but I was the one who was in denial. My weight began to drop off again and my moods and my mental state left a lot to be desired. No doubt about it I had my finger firmly on the self destruction button. My family were doing their very best to prop me up and tried to counsel me at every turn. Of course, I repelled their every attempt to turn me round. I did not care. All I wanted was the immediate fix and to hell with the consequences. There seemed to be nothing important in my life and I was letting everything pass me by. Bills became reminders became red demands. I was definitely loosing the plot and failing to see that my life was important and the well being of me was the most important thing.

One night, I was changing the wheel of my car when a guy on his way from the local pub began to badmouth me. Naturally, I resolved the matter in my usual way. I picked him up and threw him over his daughter's garden edge shouting, "catch". The boys in blue appeared and arrested him for being drunk and disorderly. We all had a good laugh at their expense. Little did I know that this was to be my last laugh for a quite a while.

Within a week I overstepped the boundaries of assault with one of my sister's boyfriends. Word had come back to me via the jungle telegraph that this nasty piece of work had been taking liberties with my youngest sister Samantha. I duly turned up to express my point of view and ended up going too far. Racked with guilt I legged it to Bristol of all places and stayed there until the middle of August working on an old power station. I began to increase the amount of alcohol I was drinking in an attempt to dilute the speed I was taking. It was like a miniature atom bomb going off in my head. My behaviour at work was increasingly more bizarre and erratic. After three or four weeks I phoned Rotherham to find out what was happening. I was told there was nothing doing so I journeyed back to Rotherham for a weekend break. My instructions were for the lads to pick me up but it was the non-hat wearing section of the police who picked me up instead. As it turned out I was so far gone with the speed that I was not interviewed for the offence of assault. A lady from the Psychiatry department of the hospital came down to the cells to assess me. My mental state was in fact worse than my drug induced state. So, I ended up in court and I was remanded in custody on the hospital wing of The Wolds Remand Centre on Humberside.

This was the one and only time that I have ever been a guest of her Majesty. I was placed in solitary for about ten days. Talk about cold turkey. I was crawling up the walls and ripping bits off my tongue with dehydration. Suddenly, the door of my cell burst open and a team of pharmaceutical jailors rushed in. Their intention was to inject me with some sedative. Memories of the lagactil squad came flooding back. My immediate reaction was to push them back through the door. They took the big hint that I had laid out and they retreated onto the landing but not before making a show of slamming the door shut with a few verbals thrown in my direction.

A couple of days later one of the inmates opened the serving latch of the cell door and passed me a drink through. Never has a drink tasted so well. I soaked it up just like a sponge in a ladies bath. This little act of humanity in such a cold desolate place meant the world to me and certainly perked my resolve up.

As the inmate was passing me my third drink one of the senior screws started to talk to me from the other side of the door and mentioned different types of medication and the effects it would have on me. I agreed to his suggestions and he calmly opened the cell door and sat down to discuss things further. Why on earth they could not have approached me in this manner straight away is a mystery to me. Here was a totally different approach consisting of humane, civilised and respectful ingredients. They had learned a lot about me but once again I had learned that no one could beat the system when the system wants to win.

They eventually let me have a more exclusive cell (sink and toilet with a space for the girlie picture) and I moved in with some glee. The downside to this move was that I had an intravenous drip in my posterior, on a nightly basis, to allow the easier dispersion of the drugs. These drugs were to settle me down and allow me to sleep. What a battle was still going on within me. I felt hyper whilst at the same time I desperately wanted a good night's kip.

Due to the ravages of my drug taking my body was deficient of the necessary nutrients for good living. The only answer was to eat well and lots of it in order to build up my strength and improve my well being. The food was served three times a day in the servery attached to the wing. One of the inmates was a complete giant of a bloke. He looked as if he wore dungarees and came from the backwoods with years of cross breeding to finalise his looks and gait. He had a habit of going to the front of the queue and helping himself to as much food as he wanted. I was starving and needed my nourishment. One day he challenged me to an arm wrestle in the recess area. Whoa. That is my game. I grabbed his arm and before his brain sent a message to his eyes to blink I had his arm down and he was defeated. He slowly dragged his feet towards his cell with the biggest sulk ever known. Guess who was at the head of the dinner queue at the next sitting?

The next day I wanted some toiletries and things so I went to the tuck shop complete with an escort to buy the necessary items. I calculated how much I owed and to my annoyance I was short of a few bob. At that precise moment my old mate Slogger came bounding through the posse and slapped the necessaries down to make up the shortfall. Despite my best attempts he has steadfastly refused to accept any payment back and just growls at me to forget it. What a mate and what a generous thing to do.

Armed with my newly purchased goodies I went back to my cell feeling more human. The meeting of Slogger cheered me up no end and before long I was making regular visits over to his area and seeing other Rotherham lads. One of the Rotherham boys was the current boyfriend of my sister Cheryl called Daz. Workouts in the gym with the boys made a change from my usual daily routine. A combination of good food and exercise began to build my body up.

A Dr. Keleman came from a Secure Unit in Rotherham to interview me. He asked me a number of questions and from the little he said I gathered that basically he was assessing my mental well being. Towards the end of that week I was told that I was due a court appearance on the following Monday. On the Friday, Big Bob and a friend of mine called Julie came to visit me. She made a joke that I had evaded jail all these years and why should now be any different. I decided to tidy myself up ready for the court appearance so I went round to the resident hairdresser who was a Londoner known as Cockney Paul. He was a religious sort of guy and would never cut hair on a Sunday. "Hello Paul", I said, "I need it doing". He was still doubtful until one of his mates related a story about how the Sheffield mob was lined up and one of them made a move towards me. He was soon hauled back with the warning, "Its J. Tune you idiot", hissed in his ear. My hair was cut neat and trim.

Monday morning arrived and I had the condemned man's last meal. Full English breakfast with extras. Just after breakfast I was told I was not going to court but that I was on my way to the Secure Unit that Dr. Keleman worked at. My instant thoughts were that I would be closer to my family and my friends. The senior screw said that I should be handcuffed but instead he chatted to me like an old mate and we shared a smoke in the van whilst driving over to the unit.

Chapter 27: Secure Unit

As soon as I arrived I was processed and shown to my bed space. A little primitive to how it is now but a bed is a bed. I looked round and immediately noticed a couple of staff from the early eighties. They were fine this time. Another ten years on and they were implementing other strategies. We had all grown up and mental health treatment had come a long way.

The second thing that happened was that I had an AIDS test. It turned out negative. This was a relief as needles were never the most sterile of things.

That night, in the sanctuary of my bed, I reflected on my stay in prison and of my life. Perhaps prison had really done me a huge favour. Although the cold turkey was painful at the time I felt within myself that I had come through the worse. It is horses for courses. Some people are cured by medicine and other methods but mine was due to the cold turkey in the stripped cell. I would not take drugs to go through that again.

The second thing I thought of was that I imagined my life as sheets of paper being thrown into two bins. One bin was marked positive and the other bin marked negative. Before long I realised that the negative bin was overflowing and the positive bin had little in it. I looked carefully in the positive bin and the top sheet had the name of my Son written large and bold. The last thing I thought of was my Son Jason laughing as he played with his toys before sleep finally captured me.

Former members of the original largactil squad were working on the unit. They, too, had come a long way in terms of patient care and understanding. No mob handed techniques and certainly no injections as an alternative. They seemed to concentrate more on one to one discussion rather than their old tactics. Their adopted system was that a patient could approach them with any problem and be met with interest and a genuine desire to help. Conversely, if any patient were walking about with their chins dragging on the floor they would usher them into a side room and have a confidential talk about anything and everything.

Despite all this I was still feeling very down and the medication had affected my zest. I was sleeping for England and I felt that I was running on empty. The harsh reality of my circumstances hit me with a rush and on one of my more lucid moments I realised that I could not have my Son see me in this state and being drug dependent. A combination of constructive counselling and my own awakening to the reasons for my remand period were a constant opposition. What I did not realise was just how ill I had become. I was literally at rock bottom for the first time in my life.

Although I did not realise it at the time the medication prescribed for me by the doctor made me very sleepy but was also slowly bringing me out of my depression. My mood was certainly fluctuating from high to low. However, it took a while before my system was in any sort of equilibrium.

My family were offering me tremendous support and my sister Marina was bringing me enough fags to keep a cross channel smuggler happy for weeks. I was that agitated that I was smoking about one hundred fags a day. The court case was still preying on my mind and I knew that I would have to go back to court at some point. But, on remand I was and I had no control over my destiny.

I befriended a guy called Ken who had passed this way before. He kept telling me not to panic and that mine was a domestic, as the police would say, and that there were others in for worse activities than mine. Samantha, my younger sister, was fond of saying that I was in there for help not punishment. Listening to these two raised my spirits no end.

Visits from Big Bob tended to rile me slightly as he would breeze in with a girl on his arm and loudly announce how much sex they had had the night before knowing full well that I was in no position for having sex metaphorically or literally. My friend Julie used to see me at the weekends and on one occasion brought me some moccasins to wear around the place. These visits by so many people including my Dad and Beano of all people are still remembered fondly by me.

Mentioning Big Bob now reminds me of a time when he said, "Considering that we are supposed to be Psychos how come that we have had more women than so called sensible people?"

Just before my twenty-ninth birthday Cheryl came to visit me bearing bad news. It turned out that her boyfriend Daz, who I been in jail with before my transfer to hospital, had committed suicide whilst still in jail. Cheryl was devastated, especially considering that Daz was the Father of her Son Kyle, and I was knocked backwards for days.

I was not allowed out for the funeral but my sympathies were well in place.

I appeared twice at the Magistrate's Court via a female member of staff who escorted me in a taxi. Both times I was in the cell area but not exactly locked up. They were still obtaining psychiatric reports and obviously I was fit enough to plea. On the second occasion the magistrates were considering sending my case to Crown Court. Other patients who had been on remand were moving on to long stay institutions and I was becoming somewhat perturbed at my predicament. Out of the blue I had the best of news concerning my situation. Apparently, for some unknown reason, my accuser had decided to send a letter to the Crown Prosecution Service withdrawing the allegations made against me. What were his motives are now consigned to history and I cheered up a bit but the case was still pending. I remained in the unit on remand and I went back to my daily round of medication, sleep, visits and grub.

The unit was in some ways like a cattle market with patients coming and going at the drop of a hat. One such entrant was a tattooed Hell's Angel look alike. He must have had some sort of reputation as the staff had doubled up when they brought him in. This was a normal staff tactic in case of risk. All the other patients backed off immediately but yours truly sat there looking at this piece of work as if he was some insignificant dropping. He ambled over to me and started to talk. I offered him a cigarette and he began to tell me about himself. He explained that he needed to wear dark glasses as he had been in solitary confinement at his place of comfort and there was a red light on all the time and it had affected his eyesight. I was not fussed about him but on the other hand he posed no threat to me. Eventually I walked off to my next port of call. After ten minutes a male nurse asked me if I knew anything about a knife that had gone missing. They had regular counts of the cutlery and one knife was unaccounted for. I was as eager as the staff to find the knife, as some part of me did not want the knife appearing in my bed space. It was like an accusation and I did not want a cloud hanging over my head thank you very much. In a flash the Hell's Angel look alike had one of my favourite female members of staff called Doreen in a non-too friendly clinch. He had the missing knife pressed to her windpipe. Although I was only a patient and should not have involved myself, my reactions being what they were, allowed me to leap across a distance and disarm this Hell's Angel. As soon as I had the knife away from her throat another member of staff helped me to pin him down on the ground until the cavalry arrived. Ian, the member of staff concerned, came to thank me most profusely and I had gained a few brownie points that day.

I suppose my macho days were not in vain and I would like to think that my actions had saved someone possible harm. The story still does the rounds in the mental health circles to this day.

I was feeling more like my normal self as the days passed after this incident. Thursday, mid December, I said farewell to staff, patients and the firm's cat as I was ready to appear in court and this would certainly be a result of some description. Just before I was about to set off the Charge Nurse came rushing down the ward to tell me that I was not required as the Crown Prosecution Service had dropped the case. My immediate discharge soon followed and I quickly gathered up all my belongings ready to go. I went to the shops first to acclimatise myself to the outside world. The sense of feeling was overwhelming and one can taste it like a sweet morsel. I returned to the unit to wait for my sister Marina and to my complete dismay who should be waiting for me but my solicitor. "Oh no", thought I, "There has been a mistake". I felt a cold knot form in my stomach. The thought that the case had not been dropped after all and that I was still due at court persisted. My solicitor had turned up to warn me that the C.I.D. had said that they had been left with egg on their faces and that I should make sure that I kept my nose clean for the foreseeable future.

With that, I climbed into Marina's car and headed for freedom.

Chapter 28: Freedom – As far the system, politics and the tax man allows:

Marina's first action was to take me round to my flat. She quite rightly decided that a low key introduction to the fundamentals of my life was the way to go. I entered my flat and looked in every room to reassure myself that I had returned home. The plan was that I would convalesce at Marina's and pick up the threads of my life piece by piece. I can't speak highly enough of the support that Marina has given me over my life but never more so than at this time. She had just met her new partner Mark and he was as equally supportive of my rehabilitation. Marina left me alone for a few hours and I realised that now freedom had come my way the world was my oyster. So, what would any man do in my situation? Go round to the pub to celebrate? Hit the town? I lay down on my settee and stayed there for two hours. This was all I wanted; the right to rest in my own place and enjoy the comforting feeling that comes with being at home.

The interludes, between staying at Marina's and being home, eventually widened to a point where I was almost ready to go it alone. One day, Marina phoned me to say that there was a bus stop outside my place and that I had to catch the bus as she was not coming round in her car for me. This is a small step for most people but for me a huge stepping stone along the road to full integration into the community.

Marina pinned a note on the back of my kitchen door containing a list of dos and don'ts.

- Obtain a passport
- Don't associate with drugs
- Don't associate with drug takers
- Do my own shopping
- Join a gym

Join a gym is exactly what I did do. Boy was I knackered. Five minutes working out and ten minutes in the sauna was the order of the day. I could not do any more than that. The medication that I was taking was not designed to make me run around like the proverbial spring chicken.

Another day, Marina, her Son Dominic and I were down town doing a bit of shopping. I suddenly handed over a wedge of notes and told Marina to buy her self a posh frock. Despite her protests I insisted. This was a way of saying thanks sis from the bottom of my heart.

The rest of my family were chipping in with help and everybody was as good as gold.

Christmas came and Big Bob invited me out for an evening with him and his lady. The meeting place was a local pub in Kimberworth that was frequented by some of the districts more notable characters and molls. Big Bob and I were enjoying a decent pint of beer and a chat when Mad Clive sidled up to us. Mad Clive was known on the drug circuit along with his rather giddy wife who had a habit of blowing hot and cold faster than the English weather. "I have a right story for you J", said Mad Clive out of the corner of his mouth. "Gasping Gaz has copped a plea for the job he did five years ago". Apparently, Gasping Gaz had gone into the police station in a state of depression and owned up to a crime that he had committed five years previous. "What ever for", I asked. "Well", said Mad Clive, "He said that it was better in jail than living with your ex- wife Sadie". I nearly died with laughing. Tears were rolling down my cheek like a cheese rolling day. Big Bob, in his inevitable way said, "There is only one thing worse than a grass and that is someone who grasses them selves up". And they called me crackers.

This laugh took me to the dawn of 1994. It lifted my spirits better than anything could have done.

I started to spend a bit of time with my friend Julie who had stood by me throughout my incarceration. She had started to talk about going on holiday abroad and this seemed to tie up with my new passport acquisition. This was a different direction for me in more ways than the obvious. We went round the travel agents in town and spent quite a while looking at different holiday locations. Eventually, we decided to go in May to Kusadasi in Southern Turkey. In between times, Big Bob was having a few domestic problems with his woman. Due to the conditions of the bail notice that he was on he was not allowed to have a drink in Rotherham. So, on his birthday in April, I took him up to Sheffield to satisfy his thirst. We had our first drink in the Marples pub in Fitzalan

Square in the city centre. Within minutes he had given the verbals to a couple of girls. They were moving onto a night club so Big Bob gave one of them my phone number with the instructions to call him.

I was putting Big Bob up at the time because of the upset over the split between him and his woman. The 'Marples' pair, and I am only talking about one of the girls, phoned me up. She asked for Big Bob but he was trying to patch things up with his woman. I did not want to land Big Bob in it so I made some excuse or other. Big Bob decided to have another go with his woman so as far as I was concerned it was fair game. When 'what a pair' phoned again she said that Big Bob did not seem interested and would I like to take her out instead. So, never one for turning a challenge down, I said O.K. My first date with Maria was in the Parsons Cross Hotel that was situated on one of the roughest council estates in Sheffield. It was the sort of place where you could order anything you wanted and it would be acquired for you at half price or less within the week.

She was of Polish descent and I descended on her 40 double C's as fast as I could. I had missed my connection with the Rotherham bus so when she asked me if I wanted a coffee I said I prefer tea for breakfast. She went upstairs and reappeared moments later wearing nothing but a flimsy negligee. Having been cooped up for four months and spending some time on rehabilitation I was ready for this. Judging by the way the way she moaned so was she. Maria had been engaged nine times before and she went into overdrive to make me the tenth. Whoa. Too much, too soon. Her over attentiveness was more of a turn-off than a welcome relief. I may have been ready for a relationship but not for being shackled. In May, I told her that I was going to Turkey with a platonic friend. We parted on good terms and kissed each other like good friends do and said our goodbyes.

Julie and I set off on our holiday and it was with a great deal of   in trepidation that I boarded the plane. My friend Julie found it amusing that the great hulk J was so nervous. The four and a half hours flight seemed to take for ever but eventually the plane landed at Izmir airport in Turkey and the warmth of the sun kissed my cheeks within minutes. I was excited as anything but at the same time I kept my emotions in check. The whole process of clearing customs, constant checking of my pockets for my passport and money, obtaining my luggage and finding the correct coach was weighing heavy in my mind. Everything had to be right and there was a level of anxiety of doing everything right. Julie held my hand and told me to sit on the coach. We arrived at our hotel and soon found ourselves in our room.

I chose the single bed nearest to the window as the heat was so intense. The holiday was one big adventure and I felt that I had put a distance between my feelings of being stigmatised and the way I was then on holiday.

Jason was never out of my thoughts and this was living in my head rent free. I do not usually allow that to happen but relationships can come and go but your children are forever. Julie kept reassuring me that one day the pain I was feeling over my separation from Jason would end and that things would be alright.

All too soon, my wonderful holiday came to an end. The hotel was non-descript and the location was not much better. That did not matter. Much the same way that people never forget their first love making it is hard not to forget the first time abroad.

In my naivety, I was foolish enough to stay in the sun too long and I ended up looking like an over done lobster. Julie had told me to use protection but to my macho mind protection meant condoms not sun cream.

Back to sunny Rotherham and back to new adventures but I was not to know that. To my surprise Samantha's boyfriend at the time had made me a pine bedroom suite and installed it in my flat. What a lovely gesture from the both of them. This was the same guy I had assaulted before my remand the year previously. Samantha had played her part in keeping everyone sweet.

I was still pursuing the court case for contact with Jason and I was unhappy at the slow progress made by the then current solicitor. Not one to be letting grass grow under my feet I changed solicitors and my new one eventually obtained for me in direct contact once per month. This meant that I could visit his Grandparent's once per month to leave money and gifts for Jason. I was also entitled to receive his school reports and photographs throughout the age of consent. Not quite the result that I was hoping for but at least it was far better than the previous slow coach had obtained for me. I never missed a single birthday or Christmas any time from my separation to the present day.

Changing solicitors coincided with a change of court welfare officer. The new guy, Adrian, has since become a firm friend of mine and I cannot praise him highly enough for the work, time and energy that he expended to help me with every facet of my life. Apart from women, Adrian was with me for quite a long time until his eventual return to the fair city of Liverpool. Well done Adrian and many, many thanks.

I was following the advice given to me to attend the out patients department and Samantha came along with me for moral support. During one of these sessions I was allocated a key worker from the community mental health team in Rotherham.

Through the periods of counselling that I received and the in depth chats that I had with my family I realised that drugs had no place in my life. My determination to cling onto normality and to be the Father that Jason would be proud of was, to a great extent, the motivating reasons. As it has turned out, I have attended eight drug related deaths over the years and sometimes I look round and ask the question 'Is there anybody left?' How many old junkies do you know I wonder? This was not for me and I made every effort to listen to the advice and recommendations that were on offer and I was equally determined to follow the directions and actions that people were laying out for me.

The realisation dawned on me that my past misdemeanours had become a stumbling block in my determination to have contact with Jason. The past is the past but this was now and soon I was receiving favourable psychiatric reports. The more I received the stronger my case would be.

My introduction to the social scene of Rotherham was still on the tepid side. I did, however, meet a girl to go sunbathing with called Jill. She said that she was from Bristol and as soon as she told me I said that I could see why. Uplifting was not the word for it. I needed someone to splash the sun cream over my back and Jill did the job admirable. We shared sun and sex in no particular order. The sharing eventually merged together one day at the house of Eddie, one of the lads off the Meadowbank estate. I knocked on his door but there was no reply. Looking round I saw a blanket on the grass next to the trees. With a grin on my face I nodded towards the blanket and Jill soon whipped off her kit and took a position as the American cops say. Sun and sex certainly came together that session and so did we. Just as the tussle was coming to an end literally, the bedroom window opened and the loudest laugh I have ever heard resounded round the estate. Eddie was screaming with laughter and he was uncontrollable. Even today he relates this story from time to time and the way he tells it is that the first thing that he saw was two white blobs going up and down faster than the hind legs of a rabbit in full flight. His only coherent comment a few minutes later was, "What a cheek".

Jill went back to Bristol not long afterwards claiming tiredness and fatigue.

Next up so as to speak was Linda-Lou followed by yet another Sandra. Two brief excursions into love but no sense of permanency.

As the autumn leaves were blowing over my shoes I had back to back court appearances over my contact for Jason. No significant progress had been made and yet again the case was adjourned. On my birthday, my Cousin Amanda and her boyfriend Anton became man and wife. Oddly enough, it was also Amanda's birthday as well. Julie and I attended the wedding and the reception that followed. During the evening I mentioned to Julie that Christmas was coming round and that I did not want the sympathy vote from the family. Everybody was bringing their kids to the celebrations and I felt that there was always an empty chair where my Son should be sitting. Julie said that she had some turbulence in her life and somehow we decided to go away for Christmas. Within days, a holiday was arranged to Palma Nova in Majorca.

Just before the holiday I was on the phone to my ousin Jackie and her late husband Snuk. We were discussing the price of a washing machine that she was selling when she said that a 'Blast from the Past' was standing next to her. As she refused to say who it was I asked her to put her on. Within seconds I realised that I was speaking to my old flame Suzanne who had departed for the Shetland Isles eight years previously. My instincts were to ask her out for a date and she readily agreed. A few days later we met up for a drink and a chat. I told her that I was going on holiday with a friend and to my delight she was there for me on my return.

This time, I was not nervous about flying and Julie and I arrived at our self-catering unit without mishap. No tinsel due to the Spanish not celebrating Christmas as we do but I was out of the way and it was a restful time for me. It was an escape of sorts from the pain of being an absent Father. We spent a lot of time wandering around and spent a lovely day in Palma, the capital of Majorca.

I met a guy whilst on holiday who was from Skegness. A distinct case of coast to coast. As it was he had suffered a nervous breakdown and was on holiday for rest and recuperation. I thought that only applied to burnt-out American soldiers not some guy from Skegness who was a fork truck driver. How I attract them I don't know. One night he invited me to a bar that was doing Karaoke. After a while he thrust the microphone in my hand and said, "Have a go". This was the first time that I had ever sung in public and what a buzz it gave me. A little thing I know but for me it was a huge step along the road to recovery.

However, all good things come to an end and on the last day of the holiday Julie and I had a misunderstanding that proved costly to our friendship for quite a while. It was case of two stubborn people clinging to their views and not conceding an inch (mm). We returned to the Capital, Palma, on the coach without a word said to each other. On the plane the stewardess asked me if I wanted ice in my drink. "No love", I said, "The atmosphere will be enough".

It took until recently for Julie and I to resume our friendship. Wasted time on my part for Julie is truly one of life's nice people. As soon as the plane touched down at East Midlands my thoughts turned immediately to the waiting Suzanne in Rotherham.

With a stick of rock in one hand and an oversize donkey in the other I knocked on Suzanne's door and switched on the grin. By the New Year Suzanne and I were definitely an item.

Chapter 29: Happy Families

Suzanne was living at East Dene at the time but her Mother lived near my flat. As far as her Mother was concerned I was the bee's knees. She said to me one day that she remembered me from my early twenties and that I looked like a gangster. What with my crombie overcoat and soft-top BMW car. "What do you mean I looked like a gangster", I replied, "I was one". Boy did she laugh. She laughed the laugh that comes with full acceptance of someone else. The Mother, Mary, used to cook me meals and we often used to call in to see her. Mary was regarded as a Mother Teresa in the district because of her tireless good deeds and support. She is still a good friend even today and I regularly pop in for a cup of tea and a biscuit to dunk.

Initially, Suzanne and I met up three times per week and due to the recovery that I was still going through it was enough. I thought the world of Suzanne and my feelings towards her were growing stronger by the day.

Suzanne had, throughout her life, her fair share of turbulence and this in turn led her to an overuse of alcohol. Whenever her perceived pressures kicked in she would resort to drink. I did not understand alcohol abuse at that time and I found it bewildering to see her drink herself to a state. The relationship was better than the drug scene could ever be and that was a motivating reason for me staying with her. There was love in the relationship and it was shared between us.

Suzanne eventually ended up in hospital due to her inability to cope with life's challenges and disappointments. Her month's stay in hospital helped her to face up to her responsibilities but as is the fact of the matter she soon reverted to her answer to problems.

One day, my sister Samantha and I went to visit her and one of the patients told us that she had been discharged. Naturally, we believed the words of this woman and left the hospital muttering to our selves. Of course, she had not been discharged and she was waiting patiently for me to appear. How can any one take the word of a psychiatric patient as gospel?

On Suzanne's discharge we decided to go to Skegness for a short break. My Uncle, known as 'Rice Pudding', took us in his car for a few bob. If he could do the job for one pound less than a taxi he would be your man. You can't blame a man for trying to earn a crust but it was said that he would take the milk out of your tea given half a chance. He has been a character down the years but not necessarily for the right reasons. When I was hung up about a girl at a later stage in my life I asked him if he would speak to her again if he were in my shoes. His reply was, "If it's meant to be it will not pass you by". This has struck a chord with me and remains one of my favourite sayings, to the ladies of course.

One day, just for a joke, I said to Suzanne that I would propose to her at the exact same spot where my Cousin proposed to his lady. This was in the middle of Fantasy Island market that was teeming with people. Down on one knee went I in a romantic gesture. There was the sound of ripping material as the insides of my trouser legs parted company faster than people in a crowded room when someone has let one go. The accumulation of Suzanne's and Mary's cooking had taken its toll. What an embarrassment. It was as if all the people in the market turned round at the same time. Minutes later I was sat on the toilet in the men's room asking Suzanne to go and buy me an XXL pair of trackie bottoms. All in all, Skegness was a memorable week for us and served a valuable purpose.

Shortly after our return I bought a Suzuki jeep which enabled me to move furniture and bits and bats into my flat. Under the guidance of my support worker Faye I embarked on a project to make my flat as homely as I could.

One of my hobbies was collecting Embassy Cigarettes focus tokens. I used to place advertisements offering so much money for so many tokens. This enabled me to obtain my television and video player at a cheaper price than going to a shop. Faye helped me to receive dues and demands that I did not know that I was entitled to. I have nothing but praise for Faye and she was instrumental in my full independence.

I had, by the end of the year, fully integrated myself into Suzanne's life and family.

The integration went as far as becoming very good friends with Suzanne's sister Dianne and her husband Des. We spent a lot of time together and these were amongst the happiest times that I have had. Dianne and Des were very good to me and I had many a nice cup of tea in their house along with good crack.

Friendship, however, can go too far at times as illustrated on the day that Suzanne and her mate Racoon took my four wheeler jeep for the day without my permission. Boy was I angry. I did not know that they had taken it and I spent the day threatening to rip the hell out of whoever had stolen my transport. When I found out the true facts I just laughed at their prank and my descent into fuming anger. Life had certainly turned the corner for the better for me to laugh at the end of the day.

Summer of that year we went to the old Butlins holiday camp at Barry Island, South Wales. Des was a drummer in a cover band and his group had a gig at Barry Island. Whilst we were there we saw the farewell tour of the seventies band The Bay City Rollers. On the first night we went straight out for a bite to eat and a drink. I was feeling tired with all the driving that I had done and decided to go back to the chalet for a kip. After a few hours Suzanne turned up and her opening comment was that the chalet was in a bit of a mess. Whilst she was doing a cursory tidy up she came across a pair of knickers. Well, it does not take a rocket scientist to guess who took the flak for that one. The chalets were a disgrace and the mattress looked like a map of England with the animal stains that had been left as a tip.

The following night, a few of the Rotherham lads, who had come down to see Des's group, found themselves being pushed around by four bouncers. I took this as an affront to all true blooded South Yorkshire men and decided to lend my weight to the argument. They soon found out what pushing meant. Needless to say, we went in the club without paying and with their blessing. Inside the club a Welsh lady came up to me and asked what my name was. I replied that it was J and Suzanne leaned across and told the lady what her name was. The lady turned round to Suzanne and said, "I am not interested in you only him".

Back at home Faye had organised a caravan for me at Cleethorpes on the Lincolnshire coast. When I asked Faye how much it would cost she said that it was just part of the service. Without further ado Suzanne and I accompanied by three of her children soon found ourselves entrenched in the caravan. Although I still pined for contact with Jason I really enjoyed the family week with Suzanne and her kids. We only had a week away as the kids were due back at school as it was the end of their summer holidays.

Sometime around October I received a phone call from my Dad in Oxford who told me that his car had broken down and that his car had been taken into a garage. The repairs were to take a week and he needed to come back to Rotherham. Big Bob and I went down to pick him up. By the time that we arrived in Oxford it was far too late to come back to Rotherham and we decided to stay the night in a transport bed and breakfast place.

We went out for the last hour and decided to go in a Karaoke bar for a drink. My Dad had grown a beard at the time and the students in the place were calling him Father Christmas. He grabbed hold of the microphone and launched into a rendering of 'Crying in the Chapel' by Elvis Presley. What a result for us. He won the karaoke competition and hopped off the stage to resounding cheers. Big Bob and I took full advantage of the evenings' first prize and drank the health of everybody. In the morning Big Bob and I were enjoying a cracking breakfast with some very tasty sausages on offer. The owner of the place, a Londoner, came in and said that some of the sausages were for the dog. Big Bob immediately said, "I am the dog" and started barking very loudly. I am still not sure whether it was one of the funniest things that I have seen him do or was just typical of him.

For my birthday Suzanne had organised a birthday treat for me. Two tickets for the Tina Turner concert at the Sheffield Arena. For transport she had asked Rice Pudding to take us. He turned up with his Thai girlfriend in a clapped out Rover car. The decibels emitted by his exhaust were worse than the speakers at the concert. His girlfriend had a squeaky sort of voice and by the time we arrived at the Arena I was ready for admission to a retreat somewhere. This was most definitely the best concert that I have ever been to and I thank Suzanne for such an inspired present.

As part of my obligations I spent some time with Adrian the court welfare officer. He suggested that I made a home video and some notes about my life and me for my Son Jason. I produced about eight sheets of foolscap documenting various aspects of my life. I jokingly said to Adrian that I aught to write a book. In 2002 when Adrian left me his parting words were that I had made jokes about writing a book and that I should carry out my threat even if I was the only one to read it.

The home video and my scribbled notes were finally delivered to Jason via Adrian as an additional Christmas present. I found out later that Jason was surprised how big I was and how pleased he was to receive the gift. He asked Adrian if it was possible to make a video of my home surroundings and this was duly done a few months later. Suzanne worked like a Trojan cleaning my flat and making it spic and span. Despite her lapses she could still produce the domestics when required.

Although I remained a distant Father in terms of the courts the videos brought us together for the first time for years.

Just after this video I happened to be in the fish market in Sheffield. On an impulse I went on the weighing scales and to my astonishment I clocked just over twenty stones in weight. What a shock to my system that was. I was twenty-five Kilograms (four stone) over my best fighting weight as the saying goes. This propelled me to join Slimming World in an effort to shed the excess poundage. A combination of good advice and long walks helped me to achieve my target within a very acceptable time scale.

Alongside this were the ever increasing visits of my Mother to my flat. This eventually progressed to an over night stay once per week. She would have her tea with Suzanne and me and I was on better terms with my Mother than I had been for a while. What I did not know was just how ill she was.

Chapter 30: The Big C

One day, my Mother let slip that she had changed doctors and was attending a surgery over in Wincobank, Sheffield. I asked why she had given up seeing her time honoured doctor and she gave me a throw away remark that the new doctor had a better bed side manner. I noticed that she had lost a bit of weight since Christmas and seemed to be eating less and less. "Have another biscuit", I would say to her. "Stop fussing, will you", was her inevitable reply. This was the way of it. She would dismiss any reference to her state of well being with a snappy retort and a dismissive wave of the hand. One day, my sister Samantha told me that Mum had had a bout of stomach pains and that she was in a lot of discomfort. When I asked Mum about her problem she just said it was a bit of indigestion and that a couple of 'Rennies' would do the trick.

A nagging doubt was flying around in my head but I could not take my Mum to task over anything so I let it be. Something was not quite right and an unwelcome feeling of foreboding descended upon me. One typically late spring morning, Samantha turned up to my flat and hammered the door for all she was worth. "What's up Sam", I asked. "Where is the fire?" "It's Mum", she blurted out. "She has been admitted to the Northern General Hospital in Sheffield for an emergency operation". Samantha, Marina and me hot footed it to the hospital and made our way round to the ward that Mum was on. Marina and

Samantha went in first and it was not long before Marina came out to tell me that it was really serious.

The surgeon had told Marina and Samantha that Mum was terminally ill and that it looked as if she had cancer of the stomach. My heart flipped. My sisters had caught up with her as she was about to go to the theatre and she gave them a wave and a smile. There was nothing any of us could do at the hospital so we went back to Samantha's house to wait for any news. Within twenty four hours we were given the full diagnosis and it appeared that she was riddled with cancer. The surgeon advised us that she had a couple of months to live and that they had done all they could.

We left the hospital for the second time in a state of complete devastation. Words could not be found to describe what we were thinking or suffering and it was one the quietist journeys that I have ever had with my sisters. It later emerged that John, my Mother's live in partner, had phoned for an ambulance during the night as my Mother was in serious pain. He did the best he could for Mother and the family accord him every respect for the care and love that he gave to my Mother.

Hopes were raised when my Mother asked for a second operation but this turned out to be a false dawn and no improvement was made. My Mother was a fighter and had been all her life but this was one battle that she would not and could not win. It is testament to her will power that she never complained about her condition. Quite the opposite really.

Within weeks, she was transferred from the hospital to St. Luke's Hospice at Dore, Sheffield. Naturally, we were fussing over her and settling her in as best we could. Someone asked me to fill the water jug up and immediately my Mum said, "Don't ask that clumsy bugger to fetch it. He will only spill it". "Yeah, right", was my gruff reply. Seconds later I tripped on the edge of the carpet and spilt some water. The laughter rang round the room and put everyone at ease.

I attended almost every day and I was forever taking someone to the Hospice with me. The relations and family friends were coming out of the wood work to pay their respects. Put both sides of the family together and there are the makings of a tribe not a family. At least they turned up and I always acknowledge that fact.

Janet, my Mum's best friend, and I used to push my Mum round to a pub that was almost next door to the Hospice. A quiet drink of the black stuff always went down well. Janet was a very good friend to my Mother and she remains a valued member of the extended Tune tribe.

Over the weeks my Mum's state of health deteriorated and she became weaker and weaker. Little things became very important and none more so than the day that we spent watching Wimbledon on television. She kept nodding off with the amount of morphine that she was taking and I held her hand whenever I could.

St. Luke's Hospice is a wonderful place that has a lovely garden for the patients to enjoy. I said to my Mum that it was like The Garden of Eden and she just smiled at my words. In my mind I was preparing my Mother for her inevitable passing.

I, on behalf of my family, offer nothing but the fullest praise for all the staff at St. Luke's and long may they offer such a retreat.

The fighting spirit and dignity of my Mum was still in place though. One day, Marina turned up with some new clothing and my Mum ordered her back to the Meadowhall Complex on the outskirts of the city with the clothes and a curt directive to buy her something that was more fashionable. A doctor brought her some pictures of Elvis Presley's mansion Graceland's in Memphis. Like me, my Mum was an Elvis fanatic and the pictures meant so much to her as Graceland's was one place that she would love to have visited.

On the fourth of August at three O'clock in the morning I received a phone call from Marina to the effect that St. Luke's had told her that um was slipping away and that she was leaving us. As my car was in the garage for repairs I immediately phoned Big Bob's Mother and without further ado she took Suzanne and I to the Hospice. I held my Mum's hand and started to sing one of her favourite Elvis Presley songs called 'Young and Beautiful'. For once, the words of a song seemed more appropriate than anything I could have said at the time. As my Mum was only fifty-two the song was a fitting requiem for her.

Later that day I kept a dentist appointment along with Big Bob and Faye, my key worker, told me at a later stage that was exactly what my Mother would have expected me to do.

A week later, on a warm August day, the preparations for the funeral had come to fruition. The funeral procession began at my Mother's house on the Meadowbank estate. It is testament to the esteem that my Mother was held in that every gateway on the roads leading to the church had someone standing there to pay their respects. The buses had been diverted and the roads were still. The church was over flowing with mourners and there were flowers everywhere. Not a sound to be heard apart from the slow crunch of the coffin bearers on the gravel leading to the porch. We took our place behind the coffin and through gritted teeth sang the family's favourite hymns. Arms folded around shoulders and little hugs were given. The Vicar gave a heart warming eulogy and mentioned close friends as well as family members. Big Bob and his Mother were duly mentioned and I took pride in that they were publicly mentioned. As we left the church the strains of 'Peace in the Valley' by Elvis Presley was heard through the loud speakers. Her coffin was placed in the same grave as my brother Dave so that she was once again united with her Son. Special guests spoke their piece at the grave side and hand shakes were offered.

The wake was held at my Mother's house and in the tradition of the Tune family Rock and Roll songs were played all afternoon and jiving was the thing to do. My Mother would have approved of the send off we gave her and I am convinced that she would have preferred us to be happy rather than be sad over her passing.

Naturally, the family were distraught but life must go on. Cheryl was pregnant and the family looked forward to the new arrival. This is the way of it. Everyone has their time and then it becomes the privilege of the next generation.

Chapter 31: The long Haul Holidays

To lift myself out of my personal gloom I booked a holiday for Suzanne and myself to Kenya. I had a long term resolve to go on safari in Africa and this seemed to be the ideal opportunity and time. At the end of September we flew out to Mombasa and stayed at Nyali Beach. We had two weeks of sight seeing, sun bathing and absorption of a different culture. The pinnacle of the trip was a three day stay at the Tsavo East and West game park in Kenya and guests at the Hilton Hotel on stilts. We saw the big five of the animal kingdom and part of Kenya has remained with me. I learnt more in two weeks in Kenya than I did in two years of studying Geography at Kimberworth Comprehensive School.

On my return from Kenya, Suzanne and I went on safari to the Angel pub in town to see the wildlife at their watering hole. Big Bob was still touting the postcard that I had sent him around the pub. "Here comes Bwana", shouted one of the pack. "Did you see any elephants then J", was the most frequently asked question. "Yeah", said I. "Big Bob is sat over there". His reply was to ask me to get the deck chair off his back.

On my first monthly visit to my Son's Grandparent's I took along a wooden carving of a Giraffe. It is to my delight that Jason still has the carving at his Mother's house. This indirect contact meant that I was now receiving more information about Jason. At long last, I felt that I was moving closer to Jason and that I was playing a role in his development. Jason's Grandmother (Anita) told me that Jason had met Will Carling, the then Captain of the England Rugby team. To my absolute delight I was given a photograph of Jason meeting Will Carling. The photograph has remained in the prime position on the wall of my lounge ever since. Every time I looked at the photograph it made me more determined than ever to make contact with Jason.

Towards the latter part of the year a couple of celebrations were going off so we decided to have a joint night out. Nostalgia revisited wasn't in it. The pop group Hot Chocolate was appearing at the City Hall in Sheffield as a follow up to the very successful film 'The Full Monty'. My Cousin Amanda and her husband Anton along with Suzanne, Big Bob and I all duly turned up to see the group. They sounded just as good as ever and to see them live was for me a huge treat. We were dancing in the aisles like re-born teenagers but what the hell. Just because you have moved on a bit does not mean that you have to be a boring b******. It was a lovely night out and it set the mood for the rest of the year. Christmas's come and go and in a blink of an eye lid another year arrived. Someone asked me what my New Years resolution was going to be. I want to go to Mexico was my reply. "Why there?" the person asked. "Why not", said I.

I had heard of all inclusive holidays and I was determined to try one out in an exotic location. My energies were spent scouring holiday brochures and visiting travel agents to obtain information.

As a hobby and for something to keep myself occupied I used to turn up to car boot sales with Suzanne's Mum and her husband Alan. Al and Mary would do some wheeling and dealing whilst Suzanne and I would sell whatever items there were to sell. Faye, my key worker, was supportive as ever about me going to the car boot sales. She thought it was very therapeutic and would help me in the long term. My life with Suzanne had well and truly settled down to a steady carry on. I had kept myself drug free for a number of years now and my drinking was almost a social acknowledgement rather than a need. It was all I wanted after the turmoil I had been in. My driving force was to keep my head and shoulders above the quagmire. As the old soldiers used to say, keep your chin above the sh** and your head beneath the bullets. Not too low but not too high.

I was now under a different doctor and he repeatedly asked me to attend hospital to give blood samples and to check up on me. Dr. Yates was a really nice bloke and he always made a point of the positives in my life. He once said to me at a much later stage that I was a shining example of someone who had experienced mental health problems and come out the other side as a positive minded person. He made me realise that mental health was an illness and not a weakness. For recovery to take place strategies need to be put in place. It was much later that I could formalise the strategies that I have employed.

As I have said, my life was going along in a steady way but on the twelfth of May I had a dramatic body blow. I was sat with Suzanne having a cup of tea at her Mother's house when to my surprise my sister Samantha turned up with her new partner Mick. She was in a very sombre mood and she told me in a quiet way that my sister Cheryl had lost her baby Son Mathew in an accident. In respect of my sister Cheryl and her children Rebecca and Kyle I choose not to go into details surrounding the loss of Mathew. Seeing the devastation caused by the loss of Mathew I do not wish to stir painful memories. It is a tribute to my sister Cheryl that despite her knocks in life she remains a joy to us all.

As a pick up for me Suzanne took me to see the group UB40 and later for a weeks holiday in the caravan that had been arranged by Faye. We took three of Suzanne's children with us, Sean, Tina and Linda. Once again, the caravan holiday proved to be a much needed escape.

Despite all the tragedies that had befallen us I was still determined to book the Mexico holiday for Suzanne and myself. As soon as the uniformed hordes went back to school we jetted off to Mexico for our two weeks of hedonistic living. During my childhood I used to look forward to going back to school after the six weeks summer holiday but in my adulthood I look forward to the kids going back to school.

Suzanne always used to say that it was the best two weeks that we ever had together. It took forever to journey there but it was fully worth it. We arrived at the Royal Decamaron Hotel in Puerto Vallarta. It was all inclusive with great facilities. It was next to the beach in a perfect location. The beach was full of locals selling their wares and it did not take long for my car boot sales bargaining techniques to come to the fore. I was looked upon as the Arthur Daley of the North by the hotel residents and they would ask me to barter for them when they wanted to buy something. Life does not get much better than a fortnight of total relaxation in exotic surroundings.

One day we went on a jeep safari with a couple from Leeds called Lesley and Martin. The journey took us to the location where Arnold Schwarzenegger made the film 'Predator'. Unfortunately for us it absolutely threw it down as so happens in the jungle. We resorted to drinking tequila and singing rugby songs. The ladies became very frisky and very drunk. I found it amusing to watch the progress, or lack of it, of all the people on the safari. Suzanne said afterwards that it was first time that she ever saw me drink more than her. It was a holiday after all said and done. The safari was a wash out but boy did we have fun. We were screaming with laughter for hours.

The hotel rooms were huge and they contained the biggest beds that I have ever seen. I used to ask Suzanne if we were spending the night on her side or mine.

It was with lots of regrets that the holiday finally came to a close but I still exchange Christmas cards with Lesley and Martin. Lovely people and I thank them greatly for helping me have one of the best holidays that I have ever had.

All too soon I was back in sunny Rotherham and back in the groove. Not long after our return there was a knock on the door and to my surprise Big Bob was standing there with Gasping Gaz of all people. Big Bob immediately explained that Gasping Gaz wanted to apologise for all the hurt that he had caused. He offered his hand but I refused to take it. I did, however, invite them inside to discuss things. When we had made ourselves comfortable in my lounge I told Gasping Gaz that I was very happy with Suzanne and that I no longer thought of Sadie in those terms. Suzanne made us a round of sandwiches and I brought out the duty free drinks that I had bought on holiday. Before long, the drink had taken its toll on Gasping Gaz and he started to slur his words. The drink loosened up his tongue and he asked me if I knew that his Uncle was gay. Suzanne suddenly said, "It is not your Uncle who is gay but his boyfriend". We burst out laughing apart from gasping Gaz. He realised that a joke had been made at his expense but he did not have the intelligence to understand how. Before long, Gasping Gaz blurted out that he had tried to change my Son's surname to his. Why this muppet told me this I do not know but the music stopped for him. I was just about to throw him out when Suzanne landed a punch that only a woman could throw. It was still enough to drop him to the floor. She grabbed hold of his coat collar and dragged him down stairs to the ground level.

What on earth he was trying to achieve I have never been able to work out. All I know is that

Suzanne is the third woman I know to knock him to his knees. What a loser. He was seen a few days later wearing more bandages than an over done Egyptian mummy. A mummy would probably be more alive than he is.

The year closed with a family gathering at Marina's house and I took time out to reflect on the year. By the time the next year had begun I was in a positive frame of mind and looking forward to whatever was coming my way.

I decided to have a mega spring clean of the flat and with typical J. Tune flair I cut a fine deal with a guy called Merlin. Not named after the fish but after Merlin the wizard due to the length of his jam encrusted beard. For the princely sum of fully decorating my flat I off loaded on him all my surplus clothing, shoes etc. I could not have done better if I had donated them to a charity shop and found my place in heaven. Why be at the back of the queue when I could be living in a newly painted flat. He did a fabulous job and left with a smile on his face and specks of paint in his beard.

An old associate of mine from East Dene, DB (aka Dog's Breath), had settled on the Lincolnshire coast with his girlfriend. Word came my way via his brother that he had split up with his partner. DB's brother and a few mates were off for a weekend visit to see him and they asked if I would like to tag along. On arrival, someone suggested that we went to a pub for a meal and a drink. During the course of the evening the pub filled up with a motley crew of lager louts. Our little group of five decided to leave the premises and continue our drinks at DB's house. Unfortunately for us we were surrounded by a substantial number of the indigenous crowd. During the melee DB was hit over the head with a bottle and slashed severely with broken glass. I managed to free myself of the crowd and summoned the emergencies services. My prompt actions undoubtedly saved DB from further injuries. He was, however, in intensive care for three days in Boston. The police managed to arrest the perpetrators of the attack and I went to Crown Court as a witness for DB. The upshot of it all was custodial sentences for the accused and a twenty thousand pound payout in compensation for DB. Surprise, surprise I have never even received as much as a thank you from DB.

Not long afterwards, Suzanne's sister Annette arrived from the Shetlands having divorced her husband and living on the edge of civilisation. She had returned to Rotherham for nostalgic reasons and immediately launched herself on the unsuspecting, unprepared surplus male population. A friend of mine, Gerry the electrician, formed a relationship with her that was more to do with feelings of the groin than feelings of love. It was not long before we became the happy foursome and drinks were on the menu. Through one of Gerry's major clients I met a youngish man called Wade. It turned out that Wade was addicted to heroin and he was in a bit of a state. Just how it came to pass I am not quite sure but Wade ended up staying at my flat for about four months. During that time I took Wade through cold turkey and a programme of detoxification. It is a measure of what I achieved with Wade that he became a plumber and is now happily married with two fine children.

His Grandfather once said to me at a later date that he was in complete amazement and admiration of how I had turned Wade round.

That year, Embassy cigarettes were still giving away focus coupons with each packet of cigarettes. On average, if someone saved four thousand five hundred coupons they could exchange them for a big screen coloured television. I decided to advertise in the local newspapers for a thousand coupons for forty pounds. As a television cost about six hundred pounds in those days and I was buying coupons for the price stated it meant that I could obtain a television for one hundred and eighty pounds. All in all, I ended providing all the family with a television not to mention a couple of profitable sales.

Suzanne and I stopped going for a drink in the town pubs and spent more and more time over in East Herringthorpe. We became members of the East Herringthorpe Workingman's Club through the guidance of my Uncle Terry and Auntie June. Every Sunday there was a live group on and this became a regular event as far as we were concerned. I drank nothing but soft drinks as I was always driving and after a while I reached the stage where I did not need a drink. My Uncle Terry eventually enrolled me in the sports section of the club and I am still a member to this day. Every year the club have a weekend away and I always enjoy the crack with the lads.

I am thankful of the friendliness and respect that Terry and June have given me.

As a warm up to my main holiday we went to a small chalet on the Lincolnshire coast. Our luck held out when Suzanne won one hundred pounds on the bingo. What a result. Go on holiday and come back with more than the spending money and costs. Pity life does not run like that all the time. Pete, Suzanne's Dad, had given the kids some spending money so everybody was a little happy bunny. It certainly put me in a good mood leading up to my thirty-fifth birthday treat.

Holidays were now becoming important to me. Whereas I had been wasting my money on drugs and chemical supports I was now diverting my money to worthwhile pursuits. It is no good dreaming about places in the world if you don't make an effort to go to them. Everything costs money and it is better to spend your money on holidays rather than some product that is likely to lead to an early death, a stay in prison or mental health problems.

My rehabilitation from being dependant on drugs to a purged sinner was now enabling me to follow my dreams and go to the places that were previously just a picture in a discarded Sunday newspaper magazine.

The holiday fund jar that was on the floor between the lounge and the kitchen was now so full that I was using it as a cheap bench weight lifting bar. A fun filled Sunday afternoon counting out the money on my bed gave me the knowledge that I had enough money to buy a Caribbean cruise and stay holiday.

Before I knew it I was wearing a gaudy shirt on board the SS Sunbird and trying to persuade Suzanne to wear a grass skirt. The first port of call was to St. Lucia. It was only when we were sunbathing on Pigeon Island did I realise just how far I had come and not in terms of miles. Although the holiday meant an increase in my waist size the sheer luxury and interest of the holiday could not be matched.

On the night of my birthday we went down to the dining room a little late and the waiter directed us to a table that was situated in the middle of the room. This was not to my liking so I quietly objected at being offered such a position. Eventually, we were invited to sit at a table for two which was very near to the Captain's table. To my surprise and joy because we were sitting at this particular table a waiter thrust a bottle of champagne in the wine cooler next to the table. He obviously thought that we were part of the Captain's table guests. Cheers everyone.

The remainder of the holiday was spent at an all inclusive four star hotel in St. James's, Barbados. The highlight of the week was watching the antics of a women nicknamed 'Park and Ride'. She was far ever dropping her bikini bottoms and squatting down on the top of one of the locals. After ten minutes of 'OOOOH Lady' she would wander down the beach and park on the top of another local.

By the end of the holiday the thought came to me that I could not think of any recovered ex-druggie who had done a five island cruise and all inclusive stay at Barbados.

With white rum regurgitating itself on a regular basis we looked forward to the Millennium on our return with a smug feeling of satisfaction and optimism.

Chapter 32: So, the Millennium changes everything? (or 3 funerals and a wedding)

The Millennium celebrations were held in the East Dene Hotel with most of Suzanne's family in attendance. Irish Molly, a family friend of Suzanne's, was the unofficial photographer on the night. Naturally, I was on some of the photographs and it was one hell of a shock when I saw the results. I looked like the archetypal darts player who is vastly out of condition. Marina came to my rescue by giving me a belated Christmas present in the form of a two weeks guest pass to a town centre gym. Donning an old Leeds United shirt and shorts that belonged to the black and white era of television I turned up for a grunt and groan session.

My first thoughts were that for a bloke like me this would be a walk in the park. After ten minutes I could not walk to the drinks fountain. I was well knackered but bells rang loud and clear in the back of my head and they were telling me that this should be part of life from now on. My two weeks guest pass became a two year membership and I began to attend the gym on a regular basis. As part of my new found fitness training I joined a slimming club and I met up with Dennis who ran the club. Under his expert guidance I managed to lose five and a half stone that year. The gym work ensured that my fitness levels rose and before long my confidence soared.

Shortly after joining the gym word came through that Mick the Bomb had died. Mick you may remember was one of my old sparring partners from my Junior School days. Mick had ballooned to over twenty stones in weight and his life style did not help when his illness came. The funeral was a gathering of many of the old faces from my youth and due respect was given to Mick and his family. The size of   Mick before he died was a further spur for me to keep with the training programme.

Shortly after Mick's funeral I received news from Suzanne's eldest daughter Zoë that Suzanne's nephew Colm had died in his sleep. This was the first time that I had heard of such a tragic thing as cot death. Due to the age of the infant I will leave you with the knowledge of his passing but not the details.

Suzanne was, understandably, very distraught and it was a while afterwards that I realised that for the first time in years it was me who was the support worker and not the one being supported.

As a pick me up for Suzanne I enrolled her at the gym. She encouraged a few of her relations and friends to join as well. This arrangement suited me fine especially as we were undertaking a joint interest.

I assumed, wrongly as it turned out, that my fitness regime would help me overcome the two tragedies that had happened. In July, my Cousin Jackie's husband Snuk was found dead. Apparently, he had been in a state of depression and he was suffering from low self esteem. A verdict of suicide by hanging was recorded and the reasons were stated. I attended his funeral along with Suzanne. Once again I stared blankly at the world whilst my mind digested the circumstances surrounding Snuk's death. Another tragic and unnecessary death had occurred.

This was the third funeral in almost as many months and I sought physical exercise as a means of relief from the sadness.

I formed new friendships in the gym and this was probably a good thing as Suzanne was more and more doing her exercising in the pub by lifting a drink to her lips. Despite my best attempts I could not pass on my good feelings to Suzanne and a gap developed between us. In between times I changed key workers and whereas I thought Faye would be a hard act to follow but Claire had her own unique attributes and we became good friends within the professional arena. She always encouraged me to attend the gym and to keep on the slimming programme. One thing she always said was that there was something in me that needed to be released for the benefit of others.

My weight was dropping off and it came at a timely moment as my sister Samantha declared that she was to be married in September. I obviously needed a suit and it was my ambition to wedge my body back in my wedding suit from 1988. A small alteration was required to the waist band and I stood in front of the mirror on the morning of the wedding admiring the svelte lines. St. Thomas's church was the natural venue for the wedding followed by an excellent reception in the Green Dragon pub, Kimberworth opposite the church. It made a change to attend the church for a happy occasion instead of the sadness of the previous visits to church.

Our holiday destination that year was Aya Napia in Cyprus. This had been recommended to me by another couple that we met in Barbados. It was a great holiday and Suzanne had never looked better. The first night on the holiday I slept on a couch in the hotel reception area. Suzanne had locked me out of the room for talking to two women in the bar area after the evening meal. She said that I had spent an age talking to these women whilst I was waiting to be served at the bar. Not because, of course, that Suzanne had gone half an hour without a drink.

Back in the gym people were telling me that I looked well with my sun tan and relaxed manner. To my surprise, an old friend from the Wingfield district of Rotherham joined the gym. On his first day he had a disagreement with someone in the changing rooms and he calmly told him to wait until he had changed before going outside with the argument. At long last, I thought, someone on my wave length in the gym. For a few weeks, Paul and I worked out together and we met up on a social level. We were, and remain so, in each other's corner and continue to be the best of pals. One day, he introduced me to a former teacher of his who had just joined the gym. "Oh", said Paul, "This is Ray Brown. He used to teach me metalwork at Wingfield School". We shook hands as you do and I thought it was good of Paul to acknowledge a teacher, but aren't all teachers soft? Ray mentioned that he was a Sheffield Wednesday supporter and to my surprise and delight we had some cracking banter for over an hour on football matters. He was definitely one of the boys from the old school and he had no airs and graces. Before long, we were working out on the weights and I was quietly impressed by how much effort he put into his work. Ray is nineteen years older than me but with the banter that we have it is more like nineteen minutes. He was working as a Design Technology teacher at another school in Rotherham and he did not know anyone in the gym apart from Paul.

Ray, Paul and me became a recognised trio in the gym and we began to join in other classes at the gym. Although I was not to know it at the time Ray was to become an integral part of my life over the next years.

At the end of the year I was presented with a shield from Dennis for being the slimmer of the year at his slimming club. My name was also the number one in the gym for reaching my target weight and fitness objectives. Ray, being Ray, asked me was the presentation in anticipation rather than for what had happened. Cheeky bugger.

Chapter 33: Another loss but they did not bury her

In February 2001, Samantha, her new husband Mick, her Son Luke and I went to the capital for the day. What a laugh. We were like silly little kids having a day out. Samantha kept going up to homeless people who were in their makings in doorways and telling them to wake up. It was good for me as we went to China Town for lunch. I had never been there before despite having worked in London for two and a half years previously. Sometimes, Samantha and I look at the video I made of that day and we still laugh at our antics.

On the back of the grand day out, I booked as usual an all-inclusive holiday in Belek, Southern Turkey. As a couple, this was to be the last time that Suzanne and I went on holiday together. It was good value for the money but the gulf between us was becoming wider. On our return I booked a holiday at a cheaper rate for Benidorm in Spain the following year. The intention was to take Suzanne and her three youngest children, Dianne and Des and their two kids plus Irish Molly and her offspring. Noah could not have taken any more.

Suzanne increasingly began to question the amount of time that I was spending at the gym. I told her that she was a member of the gym and there was nothing stopping her from going to the gym with me. My life style did not include drinking in pubs and definitely not spending time with

Suzanne's cronies. Eventually I asked her to stop drinking for a month but she never managed it. By the end of June our relationship ground to a halt. I spent some time on my own at Whitby to mull things over and I came to the conclusion that Suzanne and I were running different agendas and that our life styles were not comparable. We have remained friends and I always wish her well.

My time in Whitby was not all together wasted as I met Mel in one of Whitby's larger pubs. She had all the right ingredients, petite, blonde, blue eyes and was not in Rotherham. I could relax with Mel and for three or four months I was a regular visitor to the North Yorkshire coast. Most mornings I awoke to the sound of seagulls screeching. It was a change from hearing the sparrows coughing their way to an early breakfast. A night of passion followed by grilled kippers. It's a man's life or life for a man.

Seeing Mel was just like being on an extended holiday. Whether it was because I was away from sunny Rotherham I don't know but we perfectly matched in every department. I thought that this happiness would last but eventually the distance problem began to take its toll. Although I loved every moment I spent with her I found that I could not keep our appointments on time. So it came to pass that I received a letter from her asking why I had not written to her for a week. I had sent a return letter but this was obviously the kiss goodbye. Much later, I found out that she was involved with another guy so I left well alone. The positive aspect of the relationship was that I had put some distance between Suzanne and myself. It was Time Gentlemen Please where Suzanne was concerned and the next drink was on the bar.

Meanwhile, I started to go to an adult disco on a Tuesday night and the doorman on duty was my old mate Doug from school. "What's this place", I said, "Last Chance Hotel?" Doug just laughed and told me to get in amongst it. What a place. There was a ratio of three women to every man coupled with my type of music. I fitted the exact ingredient for the women in the place. Being male, upright, breathing with no ring on my finger and having my own accommodation. Before long, Northern Soul was playing as soon as word went round that J was in the building.

Like a kid in a candy shop I wandered round the place not knowing whom to pick. By the end of the first night I had sorted the women I spoke to in alphabetical order and went from there. By the time I reached Z I was dead on my feet not to mention other extremities. I still see some of the women from time to time and it is always laughter first, agenda second.

Just down the road from the Last Chance Hotel was another adult meeting place and it was here that I met a girl who I nicknamed Barbie Doll. She fitted my criteria right down to the dress size. We had a few trips out to sample the country air and at one point she said to me, "Must we always have sex first then a bacon sandwich?" So, from then on, we had the bacon sandwich first then the

305

afters. We did try to be romantic and not just lustful so the green and pleasant land was visited on numerous occasions. A trip to Bakewell in Derbyshire was made memorable by Barbie Doll wearing a long leather coat with just the bare essentials underneath. By the time we left Bakewell it was just the essentials underneath.

One afternoon, we were nearly run over by a combined harvester in a field in the Peak District. Such was our desire to share DNA we never noticed it. On another occasion, she left my jeep in such a hurry she dropped her bra. It was trapped in the passenger door flapping like a warning flag for hours. The entire district laughed like crazy when I drove past and parked up. I looked out of my flat window and eventually realised what everybody was laughing at. You can imagine the catcalls when I went to retrieve the bra.

The affair ended when an old friend of mine apparently told Barbie Doll that I was going on holiday with Suzanne and her family. Despite my explanations that Suzanne and I had a platonic friendship Barbie took off. Off to meet her Ken no doubt.

By the end of the summer I had befriended a guy who shared some common interests of mine. Sometimes, being nice can be taken for being soft and this guy decided to take a few liberties with me and some people who were connected to me. He was, or still is as far as I know, an alleged martial arts expert. Black belt no less as half of Rotherham had been told by no less an expert than himself. His favourite repost to any threat or insult was inevitably, "What goes this way goes that way". He decided to offend two of my nearest and thus the scene was set for a meeting at the O.K.-de-sac. As he was mouthing off and generally being a bullying oaf I stood there with my arms folded and very still. Obviously, he had not noticed that the music had stopped. As he was swaggering about like a rapper on a mission I let one go straight to his jaw. He hit the ground faster than a pine tree before the cry of 'Timber' had been uttered. I stood over the prone body and as soon as he opened one of his eyes I asked him, "If you are a black belt what Dan does that make me?" Although I was conscious that I was going in another direction well away from the fist-first mentality, there was the self-defence element against a now ex-martial arts expert. His exceptional cheap facial cosmetic treatment had slightly improved his looks but he is still referred to as Jack Palance's Dog. (Alias JPD).

Well into autumn and closing in on my birthday I decided to go to Scotland with my Cousin Bet and her husband Mac. As it happens, it was also Bet's birthday on the same day. The other guest was a friend of Bet's called Jean. We all stayed at the home of Mac's Mum. The weekend went very well with some sightseeing and relaxation thrown in. On the last night we had our birthday celebrations in the local village followed by extended socialising back at the house.

The night became noisier with verbal hostilities being exchanged between the Scots and the

English. I decided to bail out and packed my things and left. It was my intention to thumb a lift down the motorway back to sunny Rotherham. Before my thumb experienced the first pangs of repetitive strain syndrome the boys in blue stopped their patrol car and invited me to rest my weary bones on the back seat. The third degree went on for a long time and I can only assume that boredom was an occupational hazard of being a policeman in the depths of Scotland. I suppose that a man wearing a beanie hat was more of a threat than the usual suspects. The upshot of it all was that I ended up with a thirty pound fine for Jay walking.

After many goodbyes and a somewhat complicated journey I arrived back at sunny Rotherham feeling as if I had not had time away. It was almost as if my flat had become my holiday destination. No wonder people come back from their annual holidays abroad and say never again.

Yet another funeral came along on a murky cold day in December. Although I have moved on from my roots I will always pay due respect to old friends and acquaintances from the old days. One of my old friends called Harry had been fatally injured whilst walking alongside the railway track. Standing alongside me at the funeral was Paul from the gym and his partner Carol. I appreciated the respect that they paid and also the support that they gave me at such a time.

Approaching the festive run in, I was like Father Christmas dispensing kisses to all and sundry. The Last Chance Hotel was subjected to my presence and as the ladies were expecting some sort of present I did not disappoint. It was never gift wrapped but delivered on time. The list was too long to mention but eventually I cocked my hat and other things in the direction of a lady nicknamed Worksop. She was opposite to my usual tastes in that she could have been Cleopatra in a previous life. Looking at her slim figure, dark hair and sensual ways it was easy to understand why.

I used to take her to a grown-ups disco on the outskirts of Barnsley. One night, the Disc Jockey at the Robin Hood, as it is known, played a couple of Motown records. Worksop and I hit the dance floor and gave a virtuoso performance of Northern Soul dancing. The crowd loved it and before long there was a regular slot for Northern Soul music every Friday night.

Life seemed to be very good and I was having a few weeks of quiet bliss. Unfortunately, the lull was broken by news of yet another death of one of the Meadowbank crew. At the graveside, his so-called mates dropped a few suspicious packets of banned substances into the grave. I stood there to mutter my last respects in my newly acquired gym shirt. What a turn around. A decade or so ago I would have been climbing into the grave and helping myself to the manna from a chemist. Now, I was totally chemical dependant free and physically fit to boot. My health was now more important than chemically induced relief and the knowledge that yet another taker had not made it to forty reinforced my belief that keeping fit and being stable is the only way to be.

The eventual holiday to Benidorm with Suzanne and company arrived and I played the part of escort, favourite Uncle and best mate to the full. We went to the entire major attractions and, in retrospect, I am extremely pleased that I did it. Suzanne and I were non-agenda for the duration of the holiday and this arrangement suited both of us. Everybody had a good time and we remain good friends as I have mentioned before.

On my return to sunny Rotherham the atmosphere was severely warmed up by an irritated Worksop. She blazed at me that I had been on holiday with another woman and what the hell was I thinking of, going off like that? A bit rich that, coming from a woman who had a fella back in Worksop. She immediately claimed that the guy was a platonic friend who shared her house and the bills. I asked her what else he was sharing as well as explaining that Suzanne and I were merely mates. This was not what she wanted to hear and raised the sound level of the conversation. I quietly told her that I did not care for her tantrums and that I did not have to explain myself to anybody especially her. I walked away with my integrity in place and a sense of assuredness. Never one to be a bully of women and it is my intention never to be so.

Chapter 34: Beyond the Cuckoo's Nest

My key worker Claire informed me over a cup of coffee that I would be an ideal speaker for a mental health group known as Beyond The Cuckoo's Nest. As I did not know about the group I volunteered to attend their seminars and workshops to learn more about their aims and objectives. The warmth of the group and the friendliness that was offered immediately took me. As a group they are involved in work that is very close to my heart and fits exactly my perceptions of the social implications of mental health.

The Cuckoo's Nest ethos is dovetailed with my sensitivities. Everyone involved in the group from service users to staff are fully integrated in the same beliefs and ideals. I was made as welcome as an old friend the first time I observed the group. This warmth, from so many people, touched parts of my soul that I had refused for so many years to be thawed. Bit by bit, with encouragement from every direction, I contributed more and more. Eventually, came the time that I presented my first workshop. Of all things, it was at the police training college at Ecclesfield in Sheffield. Acting on the sound advice of Mary, a mental health nurse, I delivered my maiden speech. To my delight the sound of applause filled the room as soon as I finished. The question and answer session that followed helped to draw out many of the issues that I have subconsciously buried for too long. Disclosure is a valuable tool in helping metal health patients on the road to recovery. Also, it enables future and existing workers in the social field to understand that mental health patients are people with needs, with feelings and require sensitivity, not rejection.

My commitment to the group and especially the group members is beyond question. It is my fervent hope that I can continue to be involved with them for the unforeseeable future. Hopefully, the story of my life's experiences can be intertwined with my talks and presentations.

With the departure of Worksop from my social calendar I turned my attentions to a local girl who I had known of for a few years. The smile was switched on, the walk enacted and the verbals commenced.

Before long, phone numbers were exchanged and the scene was set. This, I thought, could be an interesting interlude as her background ran parallel to mine in some areas. Despite my best attempts the romance went nowhere and to some extent I was grateful that J's guardian angel was looking over my shoulder. Although I thought a lot about her it was not returnable and, as subsequent events turned out, it was probably for the best that we were not an item. 'Trouble', as I now named her, disappeared for a weekend and came back with a guy in tow. "Phew", thought I, "that was quick". In my trust of her I accepted her story that she had been without for years and was eager for the old fashion courting, wining and dining. It is clear now that she could not handle romance nor differentiate between love and lust. As I had been on the circuit for a while I was ready to come in for a pit stop but the mechanic had lost her tools.

Not one for letting the grass grow under my feet I returned to The Last Chance Hotel for a starter for ten. Doug, as usual, was there to give me a welcome slap on the back and once again the bonds of friendship came to the fore. It was not long before J was circulating amongst the chancers. Someone mentioned that a Northern Soul night was happening at the Rotherham Transport Club. A couple of days later I was talking to my Cousin Bet and she gave me the description of a woman she knew who was called Paula. As it happened, this woman went to the Northern Soul dance at The Transport Club. So, in I went, and scanned the room for a woman fitting the description that Jane had given me. I saw this petite brunette sitting on a table near the front and I immediately honed in like the bee after the nectar. Being the quiet, shy, retiring boy that I am I immediately plonked myself down and carried on talking to her as if I had known her all my life. Nice one, Tuney.

Back at the gym a list went up on the member's board as a bit of a joke of names who were interested in going to Thailand for a holiday. The laugh turned to reality when two other gym members known as Haz and Jonty said they were firm favourites to go. Job's a good one and the holiday was set. After a twelve hour flight with the added journey time in England we arrived at our hotel in Phuket. "Straight to bed?" asked Haz. "Straight after we have someone to go to bed with", I replied. We went to a nearby bar and I stood there like a kid in a toy shop. Jonty sidled up to me and asked if there was anybody I fancied. I raised my arm and pointed my finger whilst saying, "I will have you and you and you". What a start to the holiday, three women in my bed on my first night. Some say that is tall story but you, the reader, can make your own mind up.

We stayed in Phuket for five days before moving on to Bangkok. Whilst in Phuket I enrolled for a scuba diving course and as soon as I passed my basic training course I was in the deep blue looking at fish and the under side of the waves. One day we went diving at the Phi Phi Islands (scene of the film 'The Beach') and the seas were crystal blue. Not bad for a Meadowbank lad with my pedigree.

Next stop was Bangkok and the view from the Grand China Princess Hotel looked straight over the river and the city. A spot of culture was in order and we went sightseeing on both days that we were there. We stayed there for two days pottering around doing the sightseeing thing. Two days without a sample of the main agenda was just about enough for a pumped up Rotherham lad to take, so my expectations of a glowing climax to my itinerary was about to be realised with the meeting of Gorm in Pattaya. She was a delightful thirty-eight year old with the body and mind set of a twenty-two year old. Whether I wanted it or not she would massage me three times per day and she was a joy to be with. I had an unforgettable week with my exotic little bird of paradise and we certainly flew the heights. Nowadays, I would sooner make love than war and boy did I live up to my philosophy on that holiday. My only regret was that I could not bring Gorm back with me. We kept in contact for a few months afterwards but the reality of it all is that I do not make promises that I will not keep.

Our stories kept the lads back in Rotherham entertained for weeks and by the comments we were receiving there must be quite a few unhappy marriages around. Most of the crack was reserved for the sauna at the gym and the memories still have an airing every once in a while.

I had told Paula that I was going on holiday and that on my return I would take her out for a night out. We went to a well known pub in old Kimberworth village known as The Manor Barn. Whilst I was at the bar four Muppets who were associated with Trouble accused me of certain irregularities concerning Trouble's property. I walked over to Paula's table with our drinks and told her it would be just a minute. As I went back to the bar the four accusers abandoned their drinks and left the scene. This spoilt my night, especially as I was in Thailand at the time the irregularities occurred.

A week later I decided to approach Trouble's boyfriend who was employed by a nightclub as a door security consultant. As I am now in the business of using my mind and my mouth and not my brawn I assumed, wrongly, that he was of the same ilk. I tried to explain in my gentleman way that I was in Thailand at the time of the allegations and as a gesture I would help him to solve the matter. He interpreted my niceness as a weakness and summoned two other shaven headed security staff before threatening me that if it was down to me I would be well sorted. His words were, to some extent, going over my head as my attention was drawn to his three bellies that were moving around like a vibrating jelly.

Three weeks before the end of the year I was returning to my flat from a shopping excursion in the town centre. As soon as I turned off the main road into the estate, Trouble and her boyfriend, who were in their car, pulled over and started to remonstrate in my direction. I stopped further up the road with the intention of finding out what their problem was and to smooth things over. The next thing I knew he ran over to my jeep and as I was climbing out of my vehicle he hit me twice in the face. I looked at him and said, "Come on then, harder". He hit me again and I told him that he could not knock the skin off a rice pudding. I grabbed hold of him as a defensive measure and told him that he was not good enough to be a bouncer at a Mothercare shop. Holding him was similar to picking up a water melon in the supermarket. Both have a slightly hard exterior with a watery pulp underneath. After a tussle I let go of him and advised him not to come my way again. I reminded his dalliance that big and hard are not necessarily the same thing. To my total amazement and somewhat disappointment Trouble had phoned the police on her mobile phone. The police arrested me on suspicion of assault and carted me off to the police station. Despite my protestations that I was the innocent victim of a street brawl and that I had acted in self-defence I remained in the custody suite. It was much later when I was released due to my solicitor exposing huge holes in their collective testimony. The stories that they had hastily concocted did not match up and the police came to the realisation of the facts of the matter. All enquiries ceased and we were told to stay away from each other and go our sweet ways. He had squealed like a ig and sang like a nightingale to no avail. The old school just does not do grass in Rotherham.

Chapter 35: Rock 'n Roll (not quite Northern Soul though)

On a dismal night just before Valentine's Day of 2003, my good mates Ray and Paul from the gym invited me to a Rock and Roll venue at the Grange Golf Club in Rotherham. Although Rock and Roll is not my first choice in music I decided to give it a go and have an evening with the lads. Towards the end of the night I found myself having the crack with, you've guessed it, petite, blonde, and blue eyes. She asked me how old I was. I replied, "How old do you want me to be?" She smiled and I smiled even more. Naturally, there was the exchange of phone numbers and the promise of a further chat. During the subsequent phone call, it transpired that she lived very close to my Father's house and we talked the evening away. Our first date was to go for a drink to the Hind Pub in the Whiston area of Rotherham. We moved on to the Milton pub at Greasbrough for last orders. I asked her back to my place for a coffee with an added warning that she would have to trust me. Later, as I was giving Jody a cuddle, I said to her, "Before anybody else says anything I have a mental health problem". She looked astonished and said, "What sort of problem?" "Anxiety and depression", I replied. "Anxious to have your body and depressed that I can't". She burst out laughing and being the gentleman that I am I left it at that.

As the weeks went by I genuinely felt that I had found my soul mate at long last. In the gym, I always referred to her as Top Table such was the esteem that I held her in. The relationship progressed to the point where I fell in love with Jody and I truly felt that it was reciprocated. She was a true lady, who always looked like a million dollars. No raised voices, no niggles and completely supportive of the direction my life was taking me. She told me that I was a very complex person and that I aught to write a book. This was the second time someone had said that to me and I related this story to my mate Ray. He seemed to like the idea of writing a book but at that time he was very busy with work commitments. "One day", he said, "We will write the book for your Son and let the world know of you as well".

I was introduced to a lot of new friends on the Rock and Roll scene in particularly Jody's friends known as The Gang. My inclusion with such a lovely crowd of people is still a matter of pride to me. Jody proved to be an expert teacher and she encouraged me to hit the dance floor at every opportunity. Just as I thought that my moves were coming together Ray sidled up to me and said, "Move over. The gardener's come for the manure". Nowadays, he rates me as good as anyone on the dance floor. Some praise.

The Gang have an active social life away from the dancing circuit and I was privileged to be involved in many of their gatherings and weekends away. Picnics to Clumber Park in the Dukeries, Nottinghamshire, were one of our main romantic locations but our favourite spot was Chatsworth House in Derbyshire.

In the middle of August, Jody and I accompanied by a couple out of The Gang known as Pam and Colin went over to Blackpool for a long weekend. We stayed in the most abysmal digs that you could find but in a perverse way we made the best of it. The jokes about the digs kept us royally entertained long after the weekend. Whilst in Blackpool we found a bar doing sixties karaoke called Ruskin's on Albert Road. This suited us all fine and Pam, being a very good singer, made the most of the opportunity. We were as sick as a Blackpool donkey when it was time to leave despite the standard (or lack of it) of the hotel. To tell the truth, I half suspected that the donkeys were having bed and breakfast there. On the journey back we stopped at a pub in Huddersfield for a drink and Pam asked me to teach her a few Northern Soul moves. So, in the car park, I laid out a number of moves and she picked them up faster than a pigeon eating crumbs in Rotherham Town centre.

The summer was a fun filled time for me and I cherish the memories of our time together. Last thing at night I would always make a point of telling Jody why I loved her so much. As lovers do, we talked of going on holiday together and what could be more romantic than a holiday to Italy. Sure enough, we booked an all-inclusive break on the Italian Riviera.

Before the holiday came round we had a superb evening on her birthday. It started off slowly as The Gang had met in the Grange for a Northern Soul Night. However, it was wrongly advertised and it was more of a charity night than a dance. Barbara and John, a couple from The Gang, decided to go downtown with us for the evening and come back to the main dance later. The laughter, the company and the total enjoyment of the night stays clearly in my mind.

The holiday had an inauspicious start as the taxi that was due to pick us up at Jody's house failed to materialise. I bundled Jody and the suitcase into my car and roared off to Rotherham. The car was parked in a safe corner of town and we made the coach with minutes to spare. Our coach stopped in Sheffield and a group of very boisterous Afro-Caribbean girls climbed on board. They were all members of a net ball team and boy were they fun. The coach was literally rocking by the time we reached Stanstead airport. Our flight was uneventful but the beauty of the scenery was breathtaking from Genoa to our ultimate destination of Diano Marina.

As part of the all-inclusive features was a trip to Monte Carlo just over the border in the South of France. We paid our respects at the grave of Princess Grace and visited a casino. Although the place smells of money and indeed there were very expensively dressed people walking about (or should I say 'Look at me strollers') it cut no ice with me. No matter how much money they could have had, not one of them could possibly have been more happy or content than I was with Jody. On reflection, it was probably the most romantic week of my life and the feelings that I had for Jody have never been equalled

A few weeks after we had returned home, we invited Ray round for a meal and to watch the video that I had taken of the holiday. Ray arrived armed to the teeth with flowers, wine and good crack. Jody provided us with a meal to remember and eventually we settled down to watch the video. Ray commented that I looked supremely contented and that Jody and I was a couple in every sense of the word. That night served to cement my feelings for Jody.

Jody, behind my back, had arranged a surprise birthday party for me at the Rock and Roll venue that we went to. When we walked in the place was festooned with banners and balloons. All the gang were there and I was made to feel very honoured. During the evening the disc jockey asked for quiet and would I sit on a chair at the edge of the dance floor. Not wanting to lose face I sat down fully expecting a 'stripogram' or something similar. To my absolute delight an Elvis Presley impersonator came from the back room and began to sing a medley of my favourite Elvis songs. Carn, the impersonator, gave me a signed poster of himself along with an Elvis scarf.

I have seen Carn on numerous occasions and I think that he is fabulous at what he does. The night was wholly unexpected and I thank Jody and everyone who bought me a present for giving me such a memorable time.

Following the birthday evening, the Rock and Roll gang kicked a few ideas around and someone came up with a proposed visit to the Royal Hotel in Whitby to see a Buddy Holly tribute band. We decided that we would all book the weekend package and the holiday was for mid December.

A few days before the event Brian and Mary from the gang invited us all round to their house for an ironing night. I did not have a clue what this was supposed to be but I agreed to go. I was asked to bring along a white shirt and I immediately thought it was some sort of adult's pyjama night. Wrong. Brian and Mary were ironing Rock and Roll transfers onto white shirts and blouses for the Buddy Holly weekend.

The weekend arrived and we had a fantastic time. The gang all wore their 'ironed' shirts and blouses on the two evenings and all the other guests said that we looked really well. As usual, I did the videoing but took time out to impress the onlookers with my resemblance to the 'Big Bopper'. Through Jody's persuasion and encouragement I took to the floor when no other couples were dancing. There are still faint echoes of the applause that we received ringing in my ears.

Christmas eventually arrived and I found myself sitting at Jody's table with a friend of hers being served king sized portions of the best traditional Christmas fare. Previously, Jody and I had scoured Rotherham to find the exact friendship ring that I wanted her to have. To look across the table at such a woman as Jody and seeing her wearing my ring was a fitting ending to what had been one of the best years of my life so far. When people asked me what my New Year's resolutions were and what did I hope the year would bring me, I merely smiled and said I was still thinking about it. Inwardly, I thought the icing on the cake would be to see my Son again, as a Father should be allowed contact with his Son.

After much discussion and cajoling along with a degree of mental arm twisting, Ray finally conceded to be my ghost writer for my autobiography. So, on the twentieth of January 2004, Ray struck the first key of the computer keyboard. When I described the events of my birth as had been related to me he looked across at me and said, "Bloody hell. We are in for a long haul here". I just grinned at him and said that my life was not that exciting. He has continued to say "bloody hell" ever since. Not surprisingly, Ray and I have had many a good laugh when writing the book or discussing future events that were to be written about. His life has mirrored mine at times and it came as a shock to me to realise that Ray was brought up in similar circumstances in Sheffield. We used to meet up every week to write or edit the book and through our shared project our friendship grew to such an extent that Ray has become recognised as an extended member of the family.

At the Grange, Ray and I would always go outside for a breath of fresh air and for the crack.

I referred to the place where we stood as the 'Non serious Department'. It did not take long for the hangers on and those in need of free counselling to come out and off load their miseries onto us. If anyone ever asked if I was alright I would reply, "Looking round I am".

The meals continued at Jody's and an evening at Jody's bistro soon became a regular occurrence. Almost a year to the first time I met Jody, the gang organised another weekend away, this time at Scarborough, on the East coast of Yorkshire. We arrived mob handed and enjoyed a weekend of dancing, eating, and sightseeing. One of our little foibles was to hold impromptu room parties where we would descend on someone's room and have our version of the 'Happy Hour'. It reminded me of the time spent at Whitby before Christmas and I enjoyed the warm feeling that comes from being with good friends rather than associates.

Out of the blue I was invited to the Cuckoo's tenth anniversary evening dinner at a prestigious venue. As an acknowledgement of the work that I had done for the project I was presented with a certificate from the Lord Mayor of Rotherham. To say that I was proud of my achievements would be an understatement.

CHAPER 36: My Son my Son

On one of those desultory mornings that Rotherham decides to inflict on its stoic citizens I made myself a cup of tea. I sat on my balcony sipping my drink and looked across at the landscape of the green belt. My thoughts suddenly accelerated through my past but with the present clinging on. Although the past has had such an influence on the way my life has been forged there has to be a time when I needed to let go of the hand holes. The friends that I have made over the years still dwell in my heart but the realisation that I was moving in new directions settled easily in my mind. I realised that this thought had been with me for a while but I had chosen to suppress it instead of letting it rise up. No one can foresee the future but deep within me was the feeling that my life was about to change again but with added value.

My monthly visits to Jason's Grandparent's continued and news about Jason filtered through. The phone call I received from Anita asking me to see her came as some concern to me as it was only a couple of weeks since I had last seen her. I dashed over to the Grandparent's house and I was ushered inside with a grave look on Anita's face. My heart leapt as I thought the worse had happened. Anita commenced to tell me that Jason had, out of the blue, began to ask questions about me and that he wanted to know more about his roots. This in turn had caused some discord in his family home. Anita asked me to keep it to myself and not to press any buttons to force the issue. I decided that not rocking the boat was the correct course of action and asked Anita to keep in regular contact with me about the situation.

Not long after the emergency visit to Jason's Grandparent's Jody, Jonty, his partner and I went to Bakewell in the White Peak District for an organised picnic and get together. During the conversation Jody mentioned that I was nearing a reunion with Jason. I had to calm proceedings down by saying that I was optimistic enough to believe that it would be a matter of days.

On entering my flat after the lovely day out I checked my answering machine as usual and to my joy there was a message asking me to ring Anita. No sooner had she said, "Jason's here. He wants to meet you", I was in my car roaring off to the Grandparent's house. My mind was whirling with questions like, 'What do I say to him?' and 'What do I do?' In the event, as soon as I saw Jason I hugged him as only a Father can hug his Son and shared the many tears that flowed. My memories of what was said have been buried under layers of sheer emotion. It is possible to have complete conversations locked in one's mind forever as it is to harness complete happiness and store that for eternity.

His Grandparent's tactfully left us alone for a while until it was time to take him back to Sheffield. I dropped him off at Fitzalan Square in the city centre and bid him farewell until the next time I saw him. In all the excitement I forgot to ask him for his mobile phone number so I still depended on his Grandparent's as go betweens.

Over the next couple of months I saw Jason on a regular basis and it was during his main school holidays that he finally told his Mother that he had been seeing me. It was a hard decision for Jason to make and for his Mother to accept. After all, it had been fourteen years since the system allowed me my proper place as a Father in the full sense of the word.

Jason and Jody finally met and they hit it off straight away. She spoilt him a little as good people do and I felt that the pieces of the jigsaw were finally falling into place.

Jody and I went on a caravan holiday for a week at Blackpool that was broken by a return visit to Rotherham to allow Jody to care for her elderly Mother. We went back to Blackpool accompanied with Barbara and John. There was a rock and roll event taking place in the Queens Hotel and the girls were nicknamed 'The Pony Tails'.
On the last day we went window shopping looking for holiday gifts. I found myself peering into shops selling designer wear and wondering if it would be the sort of thing that Jason would like. Never was my heart so full of love. Love for a woman and love for a Son.

To my delight Jason asked if he could stay over for a couple of nights every so often. The spare bedroom in the flat was organised and became Jason's room. Jason was as good as his word.

He would sleep over and soon the flat became a family home rather than a bachelor's pad. Cheryl's Son, Kyle, made frequent visits and the Tune family took great pleasure in seeing two Cousins become good friends.

In August Jason registered for Sixth Form College and I vowed to assist him in every way possible to ensure that his studies came first. Incidentally, Jody was having improvements carried out in her house and we decided that for the time being I would stay in my flat with Jason. Jody has a heavy work load and she is committed to looking after her Mother. We still managed to have evenings out and to keep in touch via the telephone. The Rock and Roll gang organised nights out to dance venues and evening dinners.

I also organised and sold tickets for two Northern Soul nights at the Grange Golf Club and to everyone's surprise but mine the evenings proved to be a great success and they still continue to this day.

Mid September coincided with Jody's birthday and the gang met up at a well-known eatery to celebrate the event. I was on top form and wallowed in the feelings that I had for her. The night ended at Pam and Colin's place for karaoke and nibbles. These were great nights and I fully expected them to always be a part of my life.

However, enough has happened in my life for me to know that life has a nasty habit of turning on you and biting lumps out of you. A week after her birthday I turned up at Jody's house for an evening out at her friend's birthday party, armed with my camcorder and aftershave. As usual, I met her with a kiss and a cuddle but when I put my arms around her she pushed me away. She dropped the bombshell that she was no longer interested in a relationship with me and that she wanted to be on her own. I was hurt and somewhat bewildered by the turn of events. My heart had been split in two. One half filled with love and the other broken with hurt.

I rationalised over the next few weeks that life must go on and that I was important. My Son needed me more than ever and through sympathetic support from family and friends I remained strong.

Looking after number one always seemed a little selfish to me but I now realise that if you don't look after number one you are not in a position for other people to extract the best out of you.

Chapter 37: The Big Four O

My response to the break up with Jody was to look forward to my fortieth birthday. It so happened that my friend Paul from the gym was close to his birthday. We started to bounce ideas around and the base line was that we are both Elvis Presley fanatics. So, the inevitable suggestion of visiting Graceland's in Memphis bubbled up to the surface. This idea was met with full approval with me as it combined my own interests and also it was a place that my Mother unfortunately never went to. Plans were made and the holiday was booked.

In the run up to my birthday I remained good friends with Jody and we were invited to a Halloween party at Barbara's and John's. Oddly enough, I had never been in fancy dress before and felt slightly foolish being dressed up as Count Dracula. When Jody and I arrived at the party I was amazed how much effort everyone else had made. It was a terrific evening and the gang excelled themselves. Although Jody and I were no longer an item it was a great evening and I appreciated Jody's company.

Jason understood that I intended celebrating my birthday abroad and he wished me all the best. His college work was taking up huge chunks of his time but he found time to experiment with music on mixing decks with the assistance of Kyle. At the last moment, Paul asked if a couple of his mates could tag along with us on our trip to America.

Paul made all the arrangements and credit is due for his efforts and of his time.

Just before my departure to America Jody sprang a surprise birthday treat on me. She asked me to pick her up and she told me to drive. We went every way which way when she suddenly said, "Stop here". To my surprise we had stopped outside the infamous 'Baggin' club. My astonishment was further compounded when she produced two tickets for the Northern Soul Dance that was taking place there. We entered the club and immediately Jody located two of her friends who had agreed to come along for the night. What a good night that was. Jody had once again come up with the goods and proved once more what an excellent organiser she was.

Our entry to America was marred with the repetitive body and luggage searches. Finger prints, photographs, questions and searches. The only surprise was that they did not ask us for D.N.A. sample or any other type of sample. Security measures are one thing but I always assumed that the British were on the same side as the Americans. Of course, we were thrown the ubiquitous comment, "Have a nice day yawl". The irony of that comment after the rigorous encounter with the security staff at the airport was completely lost on the Americans. We all agreed it was for our benefit and that the holiday started here.

After a night's rest in a motel, our designated coach wound its way from Montgomery to our first notable destination: New Orleans. Walking round the old part of town was just like looking at old films. The buildings were exactly as I expected them to be. Of course, a walk down Bourbon Street was a must as this was the setting for the Elvis Presley film 'King Creole'. I avoided the sleazy side of the town and chose to go on a steam boat cruise. Whilst eating dinner, sailing up the Mississippi river, my thoughts turned to my childhood and the times I swam in the River Don. Enough said.

The following morning the coach set off for Memphis. Although it was a long journey I found it fascinating looking at the different sights. Red Kites landing in trees, logs floating down the river, monstrous trucks with their customised cabs and a stop off at Johnny-Be-Good's eatery in Louisiana. With the sound system on the coach blaring out 'Walking in Memphis' by Cher we drove down Beale Street eventually stopping at Graceland's. We were just in time to see the Christmas lights being switched on and stood in amazement at the colourful light spectacle. The air was filled with the strains of Elvis Presley singing 'Blue Christmas'. This really set the pulse racing in anticipation for the full day's visit to Graceland's via Sun Studios on Sam Philips Street. I went to bed that night with my thoughts racing about in my head. From Masbrough to Memphis in forty years, not quite, as tomorrow would be my birthday.

Graceland's was everything I hoped it would be and more. It was a very moving experience for me especially as Elvis had been in the background of my life. I still find it difficult to describe the sights and sounds of the place. Needless to say, I felt spiritually at home there and I could not have wished for a finer fortieth birthday.

The final part of our itinerary was a stop at Nashville, Tennessee. We had a relaxed stroll round and bought our souvenirs and trinkets before embarking for home. It was four tired individuals who eventually arrived back in Rotherham but with a satisfied feeling that comes with experiencing an achievement.

Amongst the mountain of mail that was waiting for me was an invitation for two to the Beyond the Cuckoo's Christmas dinner. I asked Jody if she was interested in going but she had work commitments and was prevented from going. My sister Samantha stepped in as my dinner companion and we had an enjoyable time with the Cuckoo's group. There was no after dinner speeches though, as we all felt that we had done enough talks in the previous twelve months.

Christmas Day saw Father and Son sitting together on this special day for the first time since Jason was two years old. Part of me had shied away from thinking what our first Christmas Day of our new life would be like. As it happened, the quietness and togetherness could not have been surpassed.

Life as a Father has not always gone smoothly but Jason is flourishing in every area of his life. We do not own our children but merely borrow them for a short time. Somewhere along the line we hope that our values are absorbed by our off-springs and that they become honourable members of society. Jason has yet to decide what path he will take but he will do so in the full knowledge that I will offer and give every support possible. As for myself I am fine tuning my life and looking for advancements especially with my work for the Cuckoo's project.

Chapter 38: Poacher turned Gamekeeper

Through my mental health contacts I became aware that STR (Support Time Recovery) jobs were becoming available. In September 2005, I applied for a position as a STR worker within the Rotherham district. To my delight I was given an interview with the Early Intervention Team in Psychosis. A few weeks later I was offered a post with the team to commence work in November.

My references from my ex-consultant and Ray Brown helped in my successful job application.

The team works with people aged between fourteen and thirty-five years old who are experiencing their first episode of Psychosis. This job specification appeals to me as I have personal experiences of Psychosis from my previous life. As my story relates, I was a young man lost in a system and now my message and actions give hope for anyone facing their struggles.

After I had been working with the team for about six months my Service Manager nominated me for the Chairman's Individual Award for my enthusiastic approach and input. At the Magna Centre, Rotherham, in April 2006, I won the first Inspirational Award to be presented. The award was made by the Doncaster and South Humber Trust and presented to me by the Chief Executive and the Chairman of the Trust.

The team provide an invaluable service that is underwritten by the service user centred approach.

At one of my talks, that I still deliver, someone said that it sounded as if I had lived five lifetimes. Drug abuse, separation, institutionalised, violence and bereavements were amongst many potential permanent setbacks. Yes, perhaps I have lived five lives but there is not one of them that I would live again. My new life is full of love and optimism. Where my life takes me is not for the knowing. One thing is for sure, if it is meant to be it will not pass you by.

Keep faith with your own determination and the goodness in life will visit you. Not everyone can come through the other door as I can testify. The trick is to never allow one's self to open the first door.

As the saying now goes 'Been there, wore the Tee shirt, done the video and now wrote the book.'

Printed in the United Kingdom
by Lightning Source UK Ltd.
117956UK00001B/46-300